Running the Tape

L. James Harvey

CROSSLINK
PUBLISHING

Run Thru the Tape

CrossLink Publishing
www.crosslink.org

ISBN 978-0-9816983-9-7

Acknowledgments

A number of people have been involved in helping put this project together and I would like to publicly thank them here. First, and foremost is, Jackie, my lovely wife of 57 years, best friend, and my editor and encourager of first resorts. Many others have contributed by reading all or parts of the manuscript and making helpful suggestions. Others have encouraged me in the project and many have prayed that the outcome would be positive and a help to others.

Among those who have helped in one way or another are Dr. Tim Brown, Bill Campbell, Virginia Campbell, Rev. Chester Droog, Dr. Daniel Harro M.D., Rev. Vern Hoffman, Dr. Henry Holstege, Don Pease, Esther Pease, Todd Ponstein, Rev. Neil Van Heest, and Edward Vermurlen. A warm and hardy thanks to all.

I would also like to thank the gifted cartoonist Randy Glasbergen for permission to use some of his cartoons in the appendix on senior humor. Randy's cartoons can be seen at: www.glasbergen.com.

Special thanks also goes to Mr. Ed Vermurlen A.I.A., NCARB, a talented Christian architect, who developed the floor plans for senior centers presented in chapter 12.

Table of Contents

Introduction

When I was in my mid-fifties I looked on retirement with some trepidation. I was concerned about possible illnesses and a gradual erosion of mental and physical capabilities. I even worried about how and when I might die. In short, I shared the concerns of many about growing older and navigating through what are often called the "Golden Years." They just didn't look "Golden" to me at the time. Now that I've lived through most of them, I can see how wrong and unnecessary my concerns were.

I've also come to see that the approach to retirement that is generally accepted in society today is totally inconsistent with Biblical teaching on the subject. The Bible does not teach us to retire at 65 and then relax the rest of our lives. Nowhere in the Bible can I find anything about retirement or spending the "Golden" years at leisure.

I've written this book to help Christians approaching the typical retirement years, and those who are retired, to see these years through the prism of the Bible and to come to see, as my wife and I have, how truly great these years can be.

A few years ago my wife and I were asked to speak to a class at our church that was aimed at helping attendees improve their marriages. In preparation my wife and I examined our own marriage, which at the time had survived for 52 years. We decided to divide our marriage into thirds and independently rate each third to see which years were the best. When we compared our ratings they were identical. We agreed the third we were in was the best, the first third came in second and the middle third was last. This didn't mean the middle third was bad. It wasn't. It just meant the other thirds were even better.

Looking at our lives we have been surprised to find that our latter years are the happiest and most satisfying. This led my wife Jackie and I to write a book about ten years ago entitled *Every Day is Saturday*[1] to share our experiences in senior living. We have been experiencing true joy in a time of life where we had expected to be wishing we were younger.

This book now chronicles another ten years of living in the typical retirement years and passes on some insights and understandings that will help all who read it realize that these senior years can truly be the best years of all. I will share how biblical teaching and modern science agree on how seniors should live, how seniors can increase both their life expectancy and happiness, and how they can make these years some of the most joyful and productive of their entire journey.

Come with me as I share what we've learned about how to "Run the race" and how to hit the finish line a winner in every respect.

- LJH

---

[1] L. James and Jackie Harvey. *Every Day is Saturday*. (St. Louis, Missouri: Concordia Pub. House, 2000).

Chapter 1 - Run Thru The Tape

Work for the Lord the
Retirement Benefits are
Out of this World[2]

One of the great metaphors of the Bible is the Apostle Paul's often used comparison of life to a running race. In Acts 20:24 Paul says,". . . *if only I may finish the race and complete the task the Lord Jesus has given me – the task of testifying to the gospel of God's grace.*" In Hebrews 12:1 we read, ". . . *let us throw off everything that hinders and the sin that so easily entangles us, and let us run with perseverance the race marked out for us.*" In 2 Timothy 4:7 Paul says, "*I have fought the good fight, I have finished the race, I have kept the faith.*" And in 1 Corinthians 9:24-27 we have perhaps the most famous verses of all where Paul says, "*Do you not know that in a race all the runners run, but only one gets the prize? Run in such a way as to get the prize. Everyone who competes in the games goes into strict training. They do it to get a crown that will not last, but we do it to get a crown that will last forever. Therefore I do not run like a man beating the air, No, I beat my body and make it my slave so that after I have preached to others, I myself will not be disqualified for the prize.*"

---

[2] All sayings at the beginning of chapters are from one of Dr. Harvey's four "701 Sentence Sermon" books published by Kregel Publications of Grand Rapids, Michigan.

It is clear that Paul thought there were lessons to be learned by looking at the sport of track. Paul would have been familiar in his day with the Olympic Games that we know so well. The first Olympics were held in 776BC in Greece, according to most authorities. Paul was highly educated and he often traveled to Greece. It is even possible that he may have attended one of the Olympic Games, which were held, then as now, every four years.

The first race to be run in the Olympics was a 600 foot sprint. In fact, in the early years it was the only race that was held. Slowly other races and events were added to the games including races of 200 and 400 meters, which still are among the most popular running events. Competition was gradually added in other events such as the javelin, discus, long jump, shot put, boxing, and wrestling. The marathon race that we often associate with Olympic running wasn't actually added until modern times in 1896.

Anyone who has served as a judge at a track meet and who has had to try and select the runners positions as they hit the finish line knows how difficult it is to determine the winner, if the race is close. This is true particularly in the sprints where several runners may hit the finish line close together straining and leaning to be the first over the line. Somewhere in track history officials decided it would be helpful to have a line or tape across the finish line so it would be easier to tell who had hit the finish line first. Thus in modern running events from the sprints to the marathon we have a tape stretched across the finish line and the first runner to break the tape is the winner.

Chapter 1 - Run Thru The Tape

Hitting the tape is the goal of every runner because it is only the winner who gets to hit it and break it. In Paul's use of racing as a metaphor for life, hitting or breaking the tape is finishing the race or the end of life.

Paul in 1 Corinthians 9:24-27 above enjoins us to prepare and live our lives as a champion runner does through extensive training and preparation. He then suggests we run our races with everything we have in order to win the prize that awaits the winner.

There is a lesson to be learned here from the sport of track that is particularly applicable to Christians and their senior years. Track coaches will tell you that for a runner to do their best and to maximize their efforts they have to run *thru* the tape not just to the tape. A good runner will not let up until they are across the finish line, and not a second before.

Runners are taught to run the hardest at two points in a race. They drive hard out of the starting blocks running as fast as they can at the beginning in order to build up their speed. Runners are then taught to run to maintain that speed; some coaches call it floating or coasting, while conserving some of their energy. They are then instructed to wait until they near the finish line to give the balance of the race the best effort they can as they drive to the tape with their final burst of speed and energy. In short, the hardest running is done at the beginning and at the end of the race, and the race ends beyond the tape not at the tape.

The problem with just running to the tape is that the runner will inevitably let up a bit before the tape because they know they have the speed to cross the finish line. Letting up near the finish line has cost many good runners first place, as a runner who didn't let up drove by them at the last second for first place. Coaches will often tell their runners to make sure they "leave it all on the track." This means the runners need to hit the tape having given the race all the energy they can muster. They are taught to go thru the tape not just to it.

Runners who try to run as hard as they can every step of the way find that about mid-race they will find their energy resources depleting. They will slow, and not have a closing burst of speed to take them thru the tape. It is in pacing himself/herself that the runner gets a maximum return on their energy resource and this allows them to finish fast. We'll explore further in the chapters ahead how this truth applies to life as well as to racing.

So how does this all relate to Christians and to the end of life? It is my contention that Christians have by and large accepted a view of retirement, and the end of life, that is not Christian and has been, in fact, imposed by a secular society. It has been accepted without thinking. It is a view that accepts the idea that we can stop running before we get to the tape and just take it easy to the finish line.

Much of this misunderstanding comes from our society and our social security system and related programs. Society says, in effect, that when we reach 65 we should stop work, relax, slow down, and enjoy the final days of our lives. That's not the message we get from Paul's metaphor about life.

In our society we have come to believe that when we reach 65 or so we have earned the right to take it easy the rest of our lives. It should be noted that when the Social Security Act of 1935 was passed we were in the industrial age and much of the work was done in factories and involved hard physical labor. We are now in the information age where most of the work is done with our minds and much of the heavy work left is done with machines often controlled by computers. The old concept of retirement is outdated particularly for Christians.

It should also be noted that when the Social Security Act was passed the life expectancy was only 62. It is now 78 and rising. One expert predicted a life expectancy of 125 by the year 2050; it's arguably possible, although the Bible says in Genesis 6:3 that our days will be limited to 120 years.

Just today in the newspaper I read about a new substance discovered in red wine that seems to improve heart tissue and extend life. Another article suggests a number of medical breakthroughs are on the way to increase life expectancy even more. In short, our society generally accepts the idea that at 65 people have the right to stop working and to live the rest of their lives at leisure. Most people in the early days did not even live to collect social security and most had jobs involving hard physical labor difficult to perform with the declining physical abilities of old age. But we are in a new age. Now people have many years still to live after 65, and the number of them is rising.

At 65 seniors today have a life expectancy of another 13+ years and this is going up. In 1900 life expectancy in the USA was only 47 years. In 100 years we have added 30 years to life expectancy. We now know that if we follow good health principles we can stay active and productive well into our 80s and beyond. How then should we use these years? When does the race end? Where's the tape? Does a Christian have the option of stopping running and walking to the finish line? I believe the Apostle Paul would say we need to run hard thru the tape and that wasting 15 or more years at leisure at the end is not a viable option for the Christian.

But don't we deserve some leisure? If we've worked hard all of our life and served the Lord faithfully, haven't we earned a rest? Don't we lose energy and physical and mental capabilities as we age? These are valid questions, and we'll deal with all of them in this book.

Paul would say, however, "Run thru the tape." He would say God never requires us to do anything that we can't do. I believe the Apostle Paul would refer us to the words of Jesus himself where in Matthew 11:28-30 Jesus says, *"Come to me, all you who are weary and burdened, and I will give you rest. Take my yoke upon you and learn from me, for I am gentle and humble in heart, and you will find rest for your soul. For my yoke is easy and my burden is light."* God's burden is light and we'll find as we explore these issues further in this book that it is in following an active Christ centered life in old age that we can prosper mentally, physically, and spiritually as never before, and have a peace and joy in our senior years that few experience.

Can anyone imagine the Apostle Paul or any of the apostles retiring? If Jesus had lived would he have retired? How about Mother Teresa, Billy Graham, or any other great Christian? Bill Bright, the founder of Campus Crusade for Christ International, died at 82 a few years ago. He died of a debilitating disease called pulmonary fibrosis which gradually eliminated his capacity to breathe. Bill hauled an oxygen tank around with him to meetings and conferences and gave stirring speeches until he was bed ridden at the end. On his death bed Bill said God had given him a message for Christian seniors as follows: *"No matter what your age or health, your loving Father has work for you to do."* Bill said even on our death beds we can pray for others. Bill Bright ran a great race right to the end. I believe he ran *thru the tape* and right into the arms of Jesus who said to him, *"Well done good and faithful servant – nice race."*

But why run hard to the end if we don't have too? I believe there are three compelling reasons. First, as Bill Bright rightly says above, if we are still breathing God must have work for us to do. God expects us to use our gifts to the end. Secondly, we will be healthier and happier seniors, if we are active and serving our God. Thirdly, we will be rewarded by God in the life beyond for what we achieve here. We read in II Corinthians 5:10, *"For we must all appear before the judgment seat of Christ, that each one might receive what is due him for the things done while in the body, whether good or bad."*

As Christians we believe there are really two judgments awaiting us at the end of our lives. One relates to salvation and the other to rewards for our works. If we believe in Jesus Christ and his atoning work, and have prayed the sinner's prayer, we will achieve salvation, but there is also a judgment about our works and rewards in heaven for accomplishments in our Christian life here.

The parable of the talents is particularly appropriate here. You'll recall in the latter part of the book of Matthew Jesus was teaching about the end times and what will happen when life on earth ends. It is in that context that Jesus gives us *The Parable of the Talents* (Matthew 25:14-30). The two faithful servants in the parable, though differing in talents (one had five and the other two), were both rewarded because they had been productive and had used their talents to produce more. The third servant buried his one talent and was punished because he had not used it in his master's interest. I believe resting on the oars, living life at leisure, and retiring from God's work after we reach typical retirement years, is the equivalent of burying our talent. We may still get to heaven but our coach will not be pleased and the rewards we could have had for eternity will be significantly less. That's why running thru the tape is so important, particularly in a society that is constantly adding time to our lives. We have the opportunity to lay up for ourselves treasures in heaven. Why not take advantage of it? I believe our heavenly coach is saying to us, "Don't leave any treasures on the table," the same as a track coach says to his runners, "Leave it all on the track."

Chapter 1 - Run Thru The Tape

The balance of this book will provide information on how to finish our races with a burst of energy that will take us thru the tape and into the arms of Jesus. Next we'll look at some other things the Bible says about old age and how we should handle it.

Chapter 2 - What Does The Bible Say?

Books Inform but
Only the Bible
Transforms

The Bible actually has a good deal to say about how we should run the race of life and not surprisingly modern science is regularly confirming the guidance the Bible gives.

In reading the Bible I have been interested to read where it says that some of the biblical figures were described as having died at a "good old age." For example we read in Genesis 25:5 *"Then Abraham breathed his last and died at a good old age . . . ."* Abraham lived to be 175. He and Sarah had Isaac when Abraham was 100 years old. Most people don't remember that after Sarah died Abraham married another wife named Keturah (Genesis 25:1) and then had six more children. He certainly lived a full life. Abraham's death at a "good old age" was a fulfillment of God's covenant with him spelled out in Genesis 15:15 where we read that God said to Abraham, *"You, however, will go to your father in peace and be buried at a good old age."*

The Bible says in Judges 8:32 *"Gideon son of Joash died at a good old age and was buried in the tomb of his father Joash in Ophrah of the Abiezrites."* In 1 Chronicles 29:28 we read the following about King David, *"He died at a good old age having enjoyed long life, wealth, and honor. His son Solomon succeeded him as king."*

So what does it mean to die at a good old age? Obviously it means the senior years are good, peaceful, active, vigorous, joyful, and healthy. How then can we also die at a good old age? The answer is also in the Bible.

One major clue we get about how to live a long life comes from the book of Deuteronomy. Here God promises a long life to those who love him and keep his commandments. In Deuteronomy 6 Moses says to the Israelites the commandments God gave him to give to the people were given (6:2), "*So that your children and their children after them may fear the Lord your God, ...and so that you may enjoy long life.*" One of the Ten Commandments, of course, has a specific promise relating to this. In the Fifth Commandment we read in Deuteronomy 5:16 "*Honor your father and mother, as the Lord God has commanded you, so that you may live long and that it may go well with you in the land the Lord your God is giving you.*"

In Proverbs we also read that it is important to keep the commands of one's father and the teachings of one's mother. It says in Proverbs 6:23, "*For these commands are a lamp, this teaching is a light, and the corrections of discipline are the way to life.*" In Proverbs 9:10-11 we read, "*The fear of the Lord is the beginning of wisdom and knowledge of the Holy One is understanding, for through me your days will be many and years will be added to your life.*" This is reinforced again in Proverbs 10:27 where we read, "*The fear of the Lord adds length to life, but the years of the wicked are cut short.*"

The Ten Commandments were given to Israel and to us to guide our behavior and to help us avoid sin. It is in following this instruction that we live lives blessed by God. When we live such lives we are blessed with peace and joy and largely escape the fear, tensions, and anxieties, which can depress the immune system, lead to illness, and often shorten a life. Sin shortens life while righteousness extends it. This is reinforced in Proverbs 21:21 where we read, *"He who pursues righteousness and love finds life, prosperity and honor."*

I believe God gave us the Fifth Commandment because he knew that if we honored our parents we would also seek to please them by living according to their advice, which in turn would be consistent with God's will. It is in living lives of righteousness that we set the basis for living life to "a good old age." It is following God's commandments and guidance for life that we avoid many of life's pitfalls and prepare for the long life that God promises. This is stated directly in the Psalms.

We find it in Psalm 92:12-14 were we read, *"The righteous will flourish like a palm tree, they will grow like a cedar of Lebanon, they will flourish in the courts of God. They will bear fruit in old age; they will stay fresh and green."* We can learn a couple of important things from this passage. First, it's the righteous that prosper. Those who follow God's will, live for him, and are guided by his principles for living stay fresh and green. Second, it is implied that the old are active, alive, and bearing fruit even at an advanced age. We can say that the righteous have meaning and purpose in life and they actively produce good works, which in turn keeps them fresh and green to the very last. Abraham, Gideon, and David were righteous and, though not perfect, stayed close to God.

In the book of Isaiah we read another statement that reflects some of the same imagery as we find in Psalm 92. Isaiah in chapter 61:3 speaks words of encouragement to the Jews and says, in effect, that if they live in accordance with God's will, *"...they will be called oaks of righteousness, the planting of the Lord that He may be glorified."* We can claim that promise also. We can be oaks of righteousness, bearing fruit in old age, glorifying God, and staying fresh and green.

One of my favorite biblical characters, who I believe epitomizes the words of Psalm 92 as well as anyone, is Caleb known as one of the two good spies sent out by Moses to study the land of Canaan. You will remember the story from Numbers 13 and 14. Of the 12 spies sent out to study the land only two, Joshua and Caleb, said that the Jews could and should, with God's help, conquer the land. The other spies said the Canaanites were too strong. The people of Israel supported the defeatists and as a result spent 40 years in the wilderness where a whole generation died off. After 40 years only two of the older generations were alive, Joshua and Caleb. They were allowed to live to enter the Promised Land because they were righteous and trusted God. Joshua was leading Israel at that time, and Caleb was a robust octogenarian.

Caleb was 85 years old when the Jews again faced invading Canaan. As the Jews were about to divide up the land by lot, Caleb reminded Joshua that Moses had promised him the hill country around Hebron for his family when they returned. Moses did this because Caleb had, *"Followed God wholeheartedly"* (Joshua 14:9).

It should be noted that the hill country was populated by the strongest fighters among the Canaanites. It was going to be the hardest part of Canaan to conquer. Joshua questioned whether Caleb really wanted to be assigned that territory, but Caleb insisted, since Moses had promised him, and it was some of the most beautiful and desirable land in Canaan.

So Joshua honored Moses' promise, and Caleb and his family were assigned the area around Hebron. Listen to the words of Caleb as he talks to Joshua in Joshua 14:10-14, *"Now then, just as the Lord promised, he has kept me alive for forty-five years since the time he said this to Moses, while Israel moved about in the desert. So here I am today, eighty-five years old! I am still as strong as the day Moses sent me out. I am just as vigorous to go out to do battle as I was then. Now give me this hill country that the Lord promised me that day. You yourself heard then that the Anakites were there and their cities were large and fortified but, the Lord helping me, I will drive them out just as he said. Then Joshua blessed Caleb son of Jephunneh and gave him Hebron as his inheritance. So Hebron has belonged to Caleb son of*

Jephunneh the Kenizzite ever since, because he followed the Lord, the God of Israel wholeheartedly."

How could Caleb at eighty-five say he was as strong as he was at forty? It was because he was righteous and he followed God wholeheartedly. Obviously Caleb loved God and trusted him without condition. He was ready to fight the most difficult people in Canaan in fortified cities at eighty-five because he was fit and he believed God was with him. Caleb was bearing fruit in old age and he was still fresh and green. What a great example of what we read in Psalm 92:12-14.

It shouldn't surprise any of us that modern science is discovering the truths that the Bible lays out for an active and productive life. If we are righteous, we are following God's guidance for living and we will stay fresh and green. It means we follow God's will for how we eat, live, love, and serve him. It means we use the gifts God has given us. It means we serve others and do good works. It means we are active, which science is affirming is a key to health. It means we have purpose in life and are looking forward to a life beyond with our Lord and Savior. It means we keep busy to the end and we run thru the tape not to it. That's what Caleb did and that's what all the other great saints of God do. When we do that then we too will die at "a good old age." I'll say more about this in the next chapter.

In the last chapter I mentioned Bill Bright. Bill and his wife Vonette founded Campus Crusade for Christ International in 1951 at UCLA. Campus Crusade now has 25,000 staff members and a ministry presence in 191 countries of the world. They also distribute one of the most effective evangelistic tools the *Jesus Film*. As mentioned, Bill Bright certainly was a righteous man who followed God wholeheartedly. He bore fruit in his old age and he died at a good old age, as the scripture promises. I'm sure Bill ran right thru the tape at his death and right into the arms of Jesus.

I believe we can all think of wonderful righteous saints in the church who stayed active and productive until they went home to be with Jesus. I remember seeing Pope John Paul II, who could hardly hold his head up, reading scripture and blessing people until he died. Billy Graham, though beset with numerous physical ailments, and saddened by the death of his beloved wife, is still, at this writing, praying, preaching, and writing. Mother Teresa was all over the world raising money for her order and working with the poor and sick in India until God called her home. They were all righteous, they stayed fresh and green and they bore fruit until the very end. They ran through the tape.

Some seniors reading this are probably thinking I don't have the energy to run that hard. We'll deal more with this later, but it must be said here that God never has unreasonable expectations for us. In Matthew 11:29-30 we read, *"Take my yoke upon you and learn from me, for I am gentle and humble in heart, and you will find rest for your souls. For my yoke is easy and my burden is light."* If we work in areas where God has gifted us, our burden is light. In 1 Peter 4:10-11 we read, *"Each one should use whatever gift he has received to serve* others, *faithfully administering God's grace in various forms. . . . . the strength God provides, so that in all things God may be praised through Jesus Christ. . . ."*

A key to successful Christian service in our latter years is recognizing what God has gifted us to do and in limiting our work for him to those areas. The wonderful Christians mentioned above loved what they were doing, their burdens were light, and they found rest for their souls. We can too.

Trying to do too much and in areas where we aren't gifted is a formula for trouble. If we are doing things we like, we will be more productive and it will be enjoyable and fruitful. Our activity, as we'll see later, will actually increase our energy and it will help keep us "fresh and green." A good mixture of work, and recreation to recharge the batteries, is a formula for long and productive life. Our senior years actually provide many of us the opportunity to take our faith and relationship to God to a new level. We can even run the good race harder at the end finishing with a burst of speed that will send us thru the tape.

If we are faithful to the end God will reward us richly. In Hebrews 6:10-12 we read, *"God is not unjust; he will not forget your work and the love you have shown him as you helped his people and continue to help them. We want each of you to show this diligence to the very end, in order to make your hope sure. We do not want you to become lazy, but to imitate those who through faith and patience inherit what has been promised."* Slowing down near the finish line out of laziness and a desire for a life of leisure isn't a viable option for the committed follower of Jesus.

Robert Clinton, a leading thinker in the area of Christian leadership estimates that 70% of today's Christian leaders do not finish well.[3] Dan Webster in his *Leadership of the Heart* seminar suggests there are three reasons for this namely laziness, sin, and discouragement. Unfortunately I believe this is true and, if so, it represents a loss to the individual as well as God's kingdom.

If there is one idea I would like readers to understand, it is that the latter years of life can be the very best, and possibly the first 2/3s of life has been preparation for the last 1/3. I believe it is entirely possible that God has been preparing you mentally, physically, spiritually, and financially to do some exciting things in his service after 65. If we stop running the race at 65, what will our "Heavenly Coach" say to us when we finish the race? I personally wouldn't want to hear it.

Now, let's take a closer look at what modern science is saying about how we should live in our senior years in order to have maximum happiness and longevity. It will be no surprise to find that modern health science is reinforcing the teachings of scripture regarding the matter.

---

[3] Wayne, Schmidt. *Lead On-Why Churches Stall and How Leaders Get Them Going.* (Indianapolis, Indiana: Wesleyan Publishing House, 2003).

Chapter 3 - What Does Science Say?

Science without Religion
Is Lame, Religion
Without Science is Blind

Whaten we look to science and the studies that have been done on aging we find, understandably enough, that science confirms completely what the Bible teaches us about aging. We find, when we sift through the evidence, that the studies we have on aging reaffirm the fact that to live long productive lives people must stay active mentally, physically, socially, and spiritually.

About a decade ago a landmark study was done with funding from the MacArthur Foundation. The study looked at all the research that had been done to date on seniors and aging and attempted to synthesize all that we knew about the aging process to that time. The study was reported in a book entitled *Successful Aging.*[4] Dr. John Rowe M.D. and Dr. Robert Kahn Ph.D. commissioned studies in a variety of areas and reviewed studies that had been done with a view in mind of finding out what factors led to successful aging.

In their book they outline the parameters of what people must do to live longer and happier. They pretty much debunk the old myth

---

[4] John Rowe M.D. and Robert Kahn Ph.D. *Successful Aging.* (New York: Pantheon Books, 1998).

that successful aging is largely a matter of our genes and our parents. In fact, they came to the happy conclusion that about 70% of the factors leading to longevity are environmental not hereditary. This, of course, means that these factors are under our control and a matter of choices we make in everyday living.

Rowe and Kahn suggest their data identified several myths about aging that were simply not true. For example they list the following six myths:

1. To be old is to be sick.
2. You can't teach an old dog new tricks.
3. The horse is out of the barn.
4. The secret to successful aging is to select your parents wisely.
5. The lights may be on but the voltage is low.
6. The elderly don't pull their own weight.

The authors are saying, based on their research findings, that the large majority of seniors over 65 enjoy good health; they can learn until the day they die; they can learn new skills, knowledge, and behaviors; their longevity is determined largely by their choices; even the sexual drive can be active and pleasurable; and lastly that seniors more than pay their own way and should never consider themselves a burden on society.

Based on the information in the MacArthur Foundation study the Mayo Clinic, the University of Michigan and other experts in the field have developed a program for successful aging called *Masterpiece Living*. This program is now being implemented across the nation in senior living communities. For example it will be fully implemented on the Breton Woods Campus of the Holland Home in Grand Rapids, Michigan in 2009.

The *Masterpiece Living Program* is founded on the principle that 70% of the factors contributing to longevity are controllable and related to the environment. The program focuses on four major areas: the spiritual, the intellectual, the physical, and the social. Seniors selecting to enter the *Masterpiece Living Program* must commit themselves to activities in each of the four areas. People sign one year agreements to follow the program. In short, the seniors agree to engage in spiritual activities such as regular Bible study, church activities, or other spiritual endeavors. They must also engage in regular program of mental and physical exercise. In addition, the seniors agree to engage in routine social activities including helping others in some way.

I don't believe it is a coincidence that the *Masterpiece Living Program* is based on principles we find in scripture for successful living and for long life. The Bible says the righteous will have long life. The righteous stay active; stay spiritually alive; serve others; and follow God's will. Science says mental, physical, spiritual, and social activity will lead to longevity. Science seems to agree with the Bible which says, righteous activity will keep us "fresh and green," "bearing fruit," and will lead to a "good old age."

When my wife and I read the book *Successful Aging,* in preparation for writing our earlier book on retirement entitled *Every Day is Saturday,* we decided to develop what we came to call

Harvey's Ten Commandments for a Successful Retirement. We based the commandments on our understanding of what scripture taught about aging as well as what science up to that time had found out about the best way to age. They are listed below. You will note they contain all of the elements of the *Masterpiece Living Program.* Here then are our *Ten Commandments for a Successful Retirement*:

1. **Be Active** – The mind body and spirit are meant to be used. Like muscles they grow and expand when used and waste away when not used. God has given us the capacity to grow. The more you use your God-given mind, body, and spirit the happier you will be. Positive activity promotes growth, inactivity kills.

2. **Exercise Regularly** – The body slows down and atrophies when it is not used. Doctors unanimously agree that regular exercise promotes both physical and mental health. As little as three 30 minute walks a week is a small investment of time, but it can yield real benefits. A more substantial program can be even more profitable. Exercise that leads to the pumping of fresh oxygenated blood through the body and brain is a wonderful healthful thing to do.

3. **Live Your Faith** – You can speak to your heavenly Father every day and hear what His words are for you – words of love and mercy through Jesus Christ. Get a good daily devotional book and use it along with your favorite Bible study guide.

Stay in touch with your Father. Attend worship regularly. Dine often at the Lord's Table. God will strengthen your faith through His Word and Sacraments. One real blessing retirement provides is we have more time to spend growing our faith.

4. **Help Others** – The joy and satisfaction you get from helping others is great medicine for your soul. Retirement is a time to give something back to your community and to invest time in volunteer activities. You will find you get more than you give because you can't "out-give" your loving heavenly Father. Helping others also strengthens our "spiritual muscles."

5. **Control Your Weight** – Excess weight saps energy, corrodes your arteries and self-esteem, and overtaxes a number of body systems. A little discipline in this area goes a long way toward increasing the enjoyment of retirement. Eat less and chew longer is a great way to enjoy food more and consume fewer calories.

6. **Have Annual Physicals** – Most serious health problems can be detected during annual physical exams. Nearly all of them caught early can be overcome. There is no better insurance for good health than to have an annual physical exam.

7. **Avoid Accidents** – Accidents that would simply harm a younger person can be a serious threat to the health of a senior. Wear seat belts at all times and take care to avoid situations where falls or accidents may occur.

8. **Be Computer Literate** – We live in an information age and no device is more important than the computer for gaining information and communicating. The computer opens a whole new world through the internet that contains endless opportunities to grow, serve, communicate, and be entertained. Don't fear computers. They are becoming more user-friendly every year. If first graders can learn to use them, every senior citizen can too.

9. **Enjoy Good Humor and Music** – There is a reason comedians and musicians have longer life spans that those in other occupations. Laughter and good music are like medicine to the body and spirit. The writer of Proverbs tells us, "*A cheerful heart is good medicine.*" (Proverbs 17:22). Good humor and good music produce a sense of joy and well-being that makes for good health and happiness. Milton Berle once said, "A good laugh is like an instant vacation." Take some of those vacations every day. We have included a section on senior humor in Appendix B so you can have a vacation or two today.

10. **Obey God's Ten Commandments** – As redeemed children of God, we know that He gave us the Ten Commandments to show us our sins but also to guide us by His grace in living a productive, Christ-centered, joy-filled life. While Christ's atoning work took the curse of sin away, the commandments

still serve as a great guide for our lives. They apply as much to seniors as to younger folks. A person living in accordance with God's will is a righteous person and eligible for God's blessings, as noted in the previous chapter.

So there you have our guide to a great retirement. It fits both with scriptural teaching and with the scientific findings from current research on aging. In Chapter 11 I will go into some greater detail on a program similar to *Masterpiece Living* that is appropriate for churches and can easily be put in place with great benefit to seniors, churches, and communities. In Chapter 12 we will look at how churches can design and develop Christian senior centers in their own facilities.

For those readers who wish to study and read more about the scientific research on aging I would suggest that you become familiar with the field of gerontology which is the rapidly growing science of the study of aging and the problems of old age. Geriatrics is the term used for the study of the physical and medical issues related to growing old.

There is a national society called The Gerontological Society of America which is a main focal point for the study and reporting of research in the field. They have a journal and an annual convention where research is reported. Their web site is www.geron.org. A good place for anyone to start studying in this field is the book mentioned earlier by Rowe and Kahn, *Successful Aging*. There are also textbooks written for courses in gerontology now frequently offered in colleges and universities across America. One of the best textbooks is written by two Christian college professors from Grand Rapids, Michigan, Dr. Henry Holstege and Dr. Robert Reikse. The title of the textbook is *Growing Older in America.*

Other agencies that contain a wealth of information on seniors include the Administration on Aging whose web site is www.aoa.dhhs.gov. This is a federal agency within the Department of Health and Human Services. The other is the National Council on Aging (NCA) whose web site is www.ncoa.org. The NCA is a non-profit advocacy agency for seniors based in Washington D.C. Appendix A contains a list of over 200 more organizations with web sites that have information that may be of value to seniors.

One increasingly finds stories reported in the press and media regarding the latest research findings on seniors. The American Association of Retired People (AARP) routinely reports such studies in their magazine. AARP is the largest organization of seniors and one of the most powerful lobbying groups in America. Most seniors will join AARP, however, you may find that the political positions they take are quite liberal and they, of course, argue for the welfare of seniors, which may at times conflict with what is best for all Americans.

A smaller organization which serves Christian seniors is called *Significant Living.* Their web site is www.significantliving.org. They provide discounts, conferences, volunteer opportunities, and a magazine.

Let's now take a closer look at the final kick thru the tape.

Chapter 4 - The Final Kick

**Go to the Edge With
God – He Will Either
Give You a Place to
Stand or Teach You to Fly**

N o racer worth their salt would slow down or stop running with one third of the race still to be run. Yet, that is what many seniors do today. They stop working for a living at 62 or 65 and assume they will live life at leisure until they die. Those who have this attitude nearly always find that leisure isn't what it's cracked up to be and science is showing us that inactivity may well hasten death rather than postpone it.

My wife and I decided to write a book a decade ago after we stopped working. It was entitled *Every Day Is Saturday.* We wrote it because we were finding that our senior years were fantastic and well beyond what we had anticipated. We titled it that way because when we were growing up Saturday was the most fun day of the week, (Sunday was the most important) and we were finding our senior days were like many Saturdays. Now, even further into this period of life, we can honestly say that these years are the best we have known. We have made and given away more money than in all our previous years, and we have served God more fully, happily, and productively than ever before. We can honestly say that this third of our lives is the best. This kick to the finish line is more fun and more fulfilling than our lives before, and that is not to imply in the least that the first two thirds was bad, it was great too.

As we look back at past years we see more clearly that every period of life has its opportunities and blessings, but each period also has its challenges and difficulties. It is no different with our latter years. While youthful energy has diminished so have inexperience and the tendency to learn by making mistakes. While energy has diminished so has the tendency to waste it and we've gained the ability to use it more efficiently. So there are tradeoffs. As we age, we find each period of life has some wonderful new vistas and opportunities as well as new hurdles to get over. If God is at the center, we can agree with the "Teacher" in Ecclesiastes 12:13-14 who says about life, *"Now all has been heard; here is the conclusion of the matter: Fear God and keep his commandments, for this is the whole duty of man. For God will bring every deed into judgment, including every hidden thing, whether it is good or evil."*

We have had a great life that has been blessed with four wonderful children and now eight grandchildren and two great grandchildren. We've had the opportunity to serve our God through teaching and serving in numerous church positions. Both my wife and I have had fulfilling professional careers, my wife's after raising our children as a stay-at-home mom. I say none of this to boast only to say that our life prior to our retirement years was wonderful, but it is still even better now. The blessings far outweigh the difficulties and the opportunities are many. Retirees can honestly say the best is yet to come both here and in the life beyond.

Mentally, physically, and spiritually this kick to the finish line is far better than we had expected. We say that acknowledging there are some aches and pains, some diminishing of physical and mental abilities, and death is ahead. We'll deal with these issues individually in later chapters, but we've come to see that running hard to the finish line will just get us to "the home office" and to God in better shape. We look forward to seeing him at the finish line.

If there's any idea we would like to leave with seniors who read this book it is that the last third of life can be the best third and that it just might be possible that God was using the first two thirds of your life to prepare you for the last third. The last third may quite possibly become the most significant third as well as the most fun and prosperous third.

Lloyd Reeb has written a book entitled *From Success to Significance*. In the book Reeb makes the case for people to consider significance as a goal rather than success, as our society defines it. Society usually judges success by the material goods, power, and status we have accumulated. A significant life is more honoring to God and is based on his judging of success rather than one judged successful by our society. Reeb's book is really keying off another book written by Reeb's mentor Bob Buford entitled *Halftime: Changing your game Plan from Success to Significance*. Buford implores people who are in mid-career and striving for success to stop and consider how they can add significance to their lives. We are saying, if people haven't found that significance fully realized in their lives by the time they stop working for a living, retirement is the time to discover it, because it is in finding the significance that one can find the full joy, peace, and blessings that God has in store for them.

Early in our lives we are generally concerned with preparing for an occupation, getting married, raising a family, and seeing to it we are successful. We easily get caught up in the routines of life and we often judge our success by the same criteria society uses. If we own a nice house in the suburbs, drive a decent car, make a good salary, send our kids to college, and avoid jail we will generally be declared successful. But God asks more from us than society does. God wants us to serve him, to love our neighbors, to do good works, to spread the gospel, and live lives guided by his spirit. He has given us gifts to develop and use in his service. We are asked to look past this life to the next and to prepare ourselves, and those with whom we have contact, for eternity. We may be running a race here but we need to see that we are on God's track team and this life is just one race. We have other races and other track meets to come in the wonderful life beyond.

Much of our success in the last third of life is related to whether we have truly identified our gifts and the mission God has for us. It may also just be that God has used the first two thirds of life to polish and hone our gifts for maximum effective use in the last third. Later in this book I will write more about this and particularly what churches and senior programs can do to help seniors zero in on their gifts and match them with programs and needs in our communities.

I believe retirement is a time to refocus, to refine, to redeploy, and to refire.

1. **Refocus** - When we stop working full time and begin collecting social security and other pension benefits we are afforded the opportunity to focus on a new phase of our life. It is important to review what we will do with it. In most cases we are looking at another 15-20 years of life. It's a wonderful gift but to take advantage of it we need to refocus on what it is God wants us to do. How has he prepared us to better serve him in these latter days?

    Many seniors will reach retirement financially secure and will not have to work. Others may wish to work part-time in order to attain financial security. In either case the time formerly used in working fulltime can be reprogrammed in new activities. Will this time be used productively or wasted? To bear fruit in old age and to stay fresh and green we must plan and refocus our time and talents on what God would have us do. A recent study found that the average senior over 65 spends 50% of their leisure time watching television. Can a Christian senior justify something like that?

2. **Refine** – The Bible teaches us that we have all been given gifts and that when we all use these gifts together we present a strong force for good. We read in Romans 12:4-8,"*Just as each of us has one body with many members, and these members do not all have the*

same function, so in Christ we who are many form one body, and each member belongs to all the others. We have different gifts, according to the grace given us. If a man's gift is prophesying, let him use it in proportion to his faith. If it is in serving, let him serve; if it is teaching let him teach; if it is encouraging, let him encourage; if it is contributing to the needs of others, let him give generously; if it is leadership, let him govern diligently; if it is showing mercy, let him do it cheerfully." In short, we as Christians are most effective when we have identified and refined our gifts and when we use them in concert to accomplish God's work here on earth.

Consider the possibility that God may want you to refine your gifts or gain some new knowledge to be used in his service. Our society now presents uncounted opportunities for learning and development. Many colleges, particularly community colleges, have free or discounted tuition for seniors who want to take courses. There are numerous opportunities to gain new knowledge and training and to use those gains in God's service. My wife decided she wanted to serve as a hospice volunteer and so entered a training program they offered at no cost. I decided I wanted to polish my writing skills so I attended some conferences for Christian writers and ordered materials that would help me. In short, if needed, there are wide spread opportunities to refine our gifts and talents and put them to work in God's service. There may even be something you've wanted to do your whole life that could now be taken up refined and applied to the mutual benefit of yourself and God's kingdom.

Some seniors take a hobby of interest and develop it in a special way. One senior I know loves to crochet. So she crochets mittens and scarves most of the year. In the fall as the cold weather sets in she donates everything she has crocheted to an elementary school to be given to children who might not be able to afford them. Another lady who loved to travel and loved children decided, after her husband died, to volunteer as a nanny for missionaries who needed someone to care for their children. She got to travel and care for children at the same time. Still others engage in arts and crafts selling the things they love to make and donating the money to God's kingdom. We can find hundreds of ways where we can use our gifts and serve God in exciting and meaningful ways.

It should be noted here that, if one is not absolutely sure where their gifts lie or what the opportunities may be for them, it is critical that you seek assistance in helping define the gifts to be refined. There are professional counselors who can help in this. Some churches may provide these resources and if not they can be found at community colleges or purchased from vocational counselors in private practice. In Chapter 11 I will mention a program called S.H.A.P.E. developed by a Christian pastor designed to help Christians define their gifts. This program is excellent and widely used by churches.

Services to delineate abilities are also provided on the internet at some sites dedicated to career development. One caution here, however, most of these sites will provide some limited free services hoping to get the individual to purchase more extensive packages. Don't get drawn into an expensive package you do not need. It is our hope that more and more churches will either individually or collectively offer these services for seniors. This will be discussed more fully in chapter 11 when senior ministry is discussed.

3. **Redeploy** – Once a senior has identified and refined their gifts they need to be redeployed in God's service. These gifts may be used entirely in volunteer service or in an activity for which remuneration is received. The gifts may be used full or part-time. The key is that one follows God's guidance and uses the gifts as directed. It is in doing this that the full benefits will be attained both individually and corporately. There are numerous opportunities to use God's gifts in volunteer services. This will be discussed later in Chapter 6 and web sites are listed in Appendix A that list hundreds of volunteer opportunities.

4. **Refire** – After you've refocused, refined, and redeployed, you can dive into the rest of your life with a new enthusiasm and fire. When we do what God asks of us, and if we are using the gifts he has given us, we not only find our tasks are fun and easy (remember he has said his burden is light – Matthew 11:30), but the rewards are out-of-this-world. Not only that but the joy we

experience serving God here makes us happier and helps keep us "fresh and green."

Dr. William H. Thomas was working with seniors in a retirement home some years ago when he discovered three plagues which he believed caused most of the suffering he saw among his elderly patients. Those plagues were **loneliness, helplessness,** and **boredom**. He wrote about this in his book *What are Old People For?* Dr. Thomas started a movement called the Eden Alternative which has developed into a worldwide association. The Eden Alternative attempts to build into nursing home procedures activities which counter these three plagues of loneliness, helplessness, and boredom. They counter the plagues by developing an environment characterized by active associations with people and animals, contact with God's wonderful creation, with spontaneous activities, with loving medical care, and by having patients involved in helping others. The Eden Alternative builds in the kind of exciting active environment that serves as an effective antidote for the three plagues. They find when this is done the patients physical and mental health improves dramatically.

A senior doesn't have to be in a nursing home to be overcome with one or more of the plagues of loneliness, helplessness, and boredom. These plagues can impact all seniors if care is not taken. The antidote for the Christian is to live an active life of righteousness. If we follow God's word and guidance, and strive to live active lives of service for him, we can have a marvelous last 1/3 of the race.

The final kick to the finish line and thru the tape can be the most fun, the most meaningful, and the most satisfying of one's entire life. God has truly saved the best until last, if we follow his lead. We can as Psalm 92 informs us *"bear fruit in our old age and stay fresh and green."* But we have to sprint to the finish line and run thru the tape. Stopping to rest and watch TV before we hit the finish line is not what our coach wants.

The Apostle Peter gave us some advice on how to live our latter days. In 1 Peter 4 after reiterating the fact that we will all face a judgment by God after death Peter gives this advice to Christians 1 Peter 4:8-11 *"Above all, love each other deeply, because love covers a multitude of sins. Offer hospitality to one another without grumbling. Each one should use whatever gift he has received to serve others, faithfully administering God's grace in its various forms. If anyone speaks he should do it as one speaking the very words of God. If anyone serves he should do it with the strength God provided, so that in all things God may be praised through Jesus Christ....."*

If anyone wants an antidote to the three plagues of loneliness, helplessness and boredom in the senior years, Peter just gave it.

So how can we take maximum advantage of our run to the finish line? Let's now take a look at some specific elements to consider in making the last third the best third.

Chapter 5 - Faith - The Force That Motivates

Faith Makes the Up Look
Good, the Outlook Great
and the Future Glorious

N o aspect of a Christian's life is more important than their faith. It should be the cornerstone of our lives. In Hebrews 12:2 we read, *"Let us fix our eyes on Jesus the author and finisher of our faith."* It is our faith that informs us about life and particularly the life beyond. It is our faith that should guide the shaping of our daily lives and the activities we choose to engage in. In our senior years our faith should become even more important to us as we prepare to meet our Lord. Often our senior years give us time to deepen our faith and walk with the Lord. If we take advantage of this opportunity, we will find our senior years are indeed our "Golden Years." If we fail to do this, these years will at best be "Fools Gold."

One of the blessings of retirement is that we have the opportunity to reallocate some of the time we spent earning a living and tending to family matters. Some of this time should be allocated to deepening our relationship with our God. Daily devotions and prayer in a time set aside to commune with God is essential. If one is already in this pattern, then the period can be extended, but if one has not regularly done this the rewards of doing it can be marvelous. Our faith can be enriched, our walk with the Lord enhanced, God's will for our lives can become clearer, and the totality of our life can take on a new luster.

We can also add to our schedules, if we aren't already doing it, a weekly Bible study with a group of Christian friends. The fellowship and learning can lift our lives to a new level.

Our faith should cause us to want to explore new avenues of service to God and his kingdom. It can be exciting to review our gifts and experiences and see how they might fit into God's plan for the rest of our lives. We may even find that the first 2/3s of our life has uniquely prepared us to serve God in some exciting new way. In the next chapter we will explore numerous opportunities seniors have to serve God and to enrich their lives and the lives of others.

One of the wonderful benefits of a mature faith is that Christians develop a "Peace at the center." This is outlined for us in scripture in Romans 5:1-2 where we read, *"Therefore since we have been justified through faith, we have peace with God through our Lord Jesus Christ, through whom we have gained access by faith into the grace in which we now stand. And we rejoice in the hope of the glory of God."*

I recall growing up that I perceived a wide difference in some of the old people with whom I came in contact. Some were grouchy and looked very unhappy while others had wonderful smiles and wrinkles in all the right places. Some looked unhappy with their lot while others seemed full of peace and joy. Why the difference? I wondered. I now believe it was their faith, or lack of it, that made the difference. G.K. Chesterton, the early 20th century English essayist, once said, "*He who has the faith has all the fun.*" How true!

For some seniors, without deep faith, every day brings them a new ache or pain, and a day closer to death. They see friends getting ill and dying. The future looks dim and the vitality and excitement of life is gone. How sad! Yet for the Christian with a mature faith every day brings hope, opportunity, and a new day of service. Even suffering and death hold out real promise and potential. Death holds no fear and, as we'll discuss in Chapter 9 just means we pass through a door and return to the "Home Office." We don't "lose friends" we just pass them on to the Lord knowing we will see them later in a wonderful life God is preparing for us.

My wife and I find, as we age, we are increasingly visiting funeral homes and memorial services for friends who have passed away. What a difference in experiences we have between those who have died without knowing Christ and the wonderful celebrations we experience when we join with the relatives of those who have gone on to the "Home Office." There's a bitter sweetness in the latter because, while the deceased will be missed, we know they are rejoicing before God's throne and waiting for us to join them for eternity.

The Apostle Paul outlines a prayer he prayed for the Ephesians that we should pray for ourselves and our friends; which sums up some of the points above. In Ephesians 3:16-19 we read, "*I pray that out of his glorious riches he may strengthen you with power through his Spirit in your inner being, so that Christ may dwell in your hearts through faith. And I pray that you, being rooted and established in love, may have power, together with the saints, to grasp how wide and long and high and deep is the love of Christ, and to know this love that surpasses knowledge – that you may be filled to the measure of all the fullness of God."*

Wow! What a wonderful prayer – and promise! We can have that if we but ask. If our lives are rooted and grounded in Christ, he will live in us and we can experience the joy, peace, and fullness of life he has for us.

As seniors we can take the advice of the Apostle Peter who in 2 Peter 1:5-8 says, *"For this very reason, make every effort to add to your faith goodness, and to goodness, knowledge; and to knowledge self-control; and to self-control, perseverance, and to perseverance godliness; and to godliness brotherly kindness; and to brotherly kindliness, love. For if you possess these qualities in increasing measure, they will keep you from being ineffective and unproductive in your knowledge of our Lord Jesus Christ."* So Peter gives us a blueprint of how to grow in our faith and service to God. And in our senior years we have the time to form and shape our faith for eternity because what we do in this life will impact our lives in the next life, as well as here.

How do we go about developing a mature faith? We attend worship regularly, we practice daily devotions, we attend a Bible study group, we converse regularly with God in prayer, we socialize with those who are mature in the faith, and we regularly practice our faith

44

by serving others. It is in the latter that we increase our "spiritual muscles." The beauty of growing in the faith is that we can continually grow, no matter what our age, and we can increase our joy and peace until the day we die, when it will explode into the life beyond. It's no surprise that those wonderful older seniors who loved the Lord, I saw as a child, had those marvelous smiling faces with all the wrinkles in the right places.

For many seniors, who have before retirement been involved in the routine activities of making a living, raising a family etc., the "Golden Years" provide them the opportunity to enter full time Christian service. Paid or volunteer service in the church or numerous charitable religious organizations full or part-time can give one the satisfaction of serving our Lord in a way not often possible before retirement. The rewards can be wonderful.

In summary, our senior years present us the opportunity in a new and wonderful way to develop and deepen our faith and walk with the Lord. It also presents the opportunity to allow that faith to guide our activities and energy into service for God, as never before. It's a win-win proposition and allows us to serve God until we take our final breath here. Let's now take a look at what some of these areas of service might be and how the activity can benefit us in many ways.

Chapter 6 - Activity - From Rest to Relevancy

Apart From God
Every Activity is
A Passing Whiff of
Insignificance

Before discussing some of the wonderful opportunities seniors have to serve God and others, there are two principles that need to be stressed. The first is that activity is essential to a healthy life and the second is that our time on earth is limited and one day we will be held accountable for how we have used it.

In Psalm 139:14 the Psalmist says, *"I praise you for I am fearfully and wonderfully made...."* Modern science is still discovering the wonders of how the human body and mind work. We are truly wonders of God's creation. One of the principles behind our existence is, however, that we were designed by our creator to be active – our bodies and minds were developed to be used. As we will discuss more fully in the next chapter, our health and well being depend on our being active and in using the gifts God has given us. We are made so that *what we don't use we lose.*

We know that if we don't use our muscles they atrophy. We also know that the more we use our muscles the greater capacity they develop, as any body builder will testify. We also have evidence that the more we use our minds, and grow in knowledge, the greater our capacity becomes to learn. The good news we are learning from those who do research with seniors is that our capacities to build muscle mass and learn seem to be present until the day we die no matter what our age. It's true our capacities diminish some with age but the potential to improve our physical and mental capabilities, absent disease, is present to the end of our lives. The good news is that seniors can grow mentally, physically, and spiritually right thru the tape and into eternity.

It seems our creator built into these marvelous bodies of ours the kind of maintenance systems we need to stay healthy. I believe it is a truism that everything God created was created good, healthy, and intended to continue in health. It is only when sin, disease, and inactivity enter that health is challenged. The maintenance systems in us, which God created, can provide health; however, they can only function if we are active.

One example should suffice to prove this point. When I was younger and people would have surgery they were instructed to stay in bed until they were largely healed. They would then be gradually allowed to get up and over a period of time return to normal activity. Today many surgeries are done on an out-patient basis and people are sent home to resume normal activity as soon as possible. Even people who have major surgery are often encouraged to get out of bed the next day and to resume as much physical activity as they can as soon as possible. Why the change in approach? Medical science learned that healing is promoted through activity. With the new approach the muscles do not atrophy from lack of use, the circulatory system is stimulated, and the bodies healing properties are maximized.

In Chapter 2 we quoted Psalm 92:12-14 where the Psalmist said, *"The righteous........will bear fruit in old age, they will stay fresh and green."* The reason the righteous stay fresh and green in old age is because they are active and constantly "bearing fruit." There you very simply have the secret to a happy and healthy last 1/3 of life. Be righteous, serve God, stay active, and you will stay "fresh and green."

The second principle of importance relates to the issue of time. The Psalmist says in Psalm 39:4, *"Lord remind me how brief my time on earth will be. Remind me that our days are numbered, and my life is fleeting away"* (NLT). Our days are numbered and the time we have on earth is precious and fleeting away. One day we will have to give account for how we used the time God has given us. When God asks us how we used the last 1/3 of our lives what will we be able to say?

Society says to us that we should retire, that we've earned the right to relax and take it easy the rest of our lives. Is that God's message? Simply put, no. Does God want us to continue working as long as we can? I doubt that too. The premise of this book is that when you cease working or reach the typical retirement age God has a wonderful plan for you to use your knowledge, experience, and gifts in some exciting and stimulating ways that can serve him and others and that will keep you, "fresh and green." It is not only possible but very likely that, if we are sensitized to God's will for our lives, the last 1/3 of our lives can be the most productive, most fun, and most exciting years of all. It would be a tragedy for the Christian to think, as our society generally does, that these years should be spent in leisure and self gratification. Who would want to stand before God and try to explain that the last 1/3 of their life was largely spent playing golf, fishing, laying on the beach, and watching TV? Frankly trying to do that would scare me.

Our society says the retirement years should be used to rest and relax; after all we have earned it through a life of work. God says be active and relevant and I'll keep you healthy and happy. One's retirement can be rest or relevance and focus on success or significance. We have a choice to make.

Does the above mean we can't do any of the leisure things we like? Of course not, it simply means we must keep a balance and use leisure to re-create ourselves not wreck-create ourselves. Too much of a good thing, even golf, can be boring and counterproductive. We need rest and refreshment to revitalize our minds and bodies, but this re-creation should be a means to an end not the end itself. Even Jesus often went apart from his followers to rest, to pray, and to gain new energy to carry out his mission.

One of the more significant recent studies on older Americans is entitled, *Older Americans 2008: Key Indicators of Well-Being*. This study, a cooperative effort of 15 Federal agencies that collect data on seniors, summarizes data from many different sources. One of the findings of this study is that on the average day those 65 and older spend at least half of their leisure time watching TV. Now, I know there are some educational things on TV but 50% sounds excessive. Are we becoming a nation of "couch potatoes?" The same study also indicates that 31% of those 65 and older are obese – not just over-weight, but obese. Is there a relationship between these figures? I believe there is. More about the weight matter will be covered in the chapter on health, but can any Christian justify spending half of his/her leisure time in front of the TV? I doubt it.

As we grow older, we need a bit more rest, sleep, leisure, and recreation to regain our energy so we should adapt to that. We should also look for activities that might serve God's kingdom and recharge the batteries at the same time. Activities like that are win-win situations. For example, if you like to play chess, you might find a person in a nursing home with whom you could visit and play chess. You help them with a visit while you enjoy doing something you like and that will benefit both of you. Others with talents, skills, and/or hobbies they could share with others might find wonderful opportunities to serve and recreate at the same time.

In the next chapter I will deal more with physical activity to keep the body healthy and fit. Let's here take a look at the mental and service activities that can help keep seniors "fresh and green."

First, let me say a word about computers. We are in the information age and the device through which much of that information passes is the computer. A computer tied to the internet opens up a whole new world of information and mental activity that seniors can't afford to miss.

I find some seniors are afraid to learn how to use a computer for fear they can't do it. Other seniors love their computers and are on them for hours every day. Computers are becoming more user friendly all the time and their use is becoming less expensive. I would encourage every senior to learn to use a computer. If children in the first grade can use them, seniors certainly can learn as well, and I should gently remind those who fear computers that fear is not a godly attribute.

Having a computer and a connection to the internet allows one to send e-mail to anyone in the world without cost or postage. It allows one access to information you can't dream of. You have access to hundreds of newspapers worldwide every day, most at no cost. I happen to enjoy reading the Jerusalem Post every day to get fresh information on Israel. I also skim the *New York Times, Washington Post*, and *Detroit Free Press* every day. As a writer, I can sit in my home office, and through the internet, actually have access to more information more easily than if I were in the Library of Congress in Washington D.C., where I used to do research. The computer gives one access to books of all types, to movies, TV programs, and information of all sorts. One can play chess or other games with people in other countries and communicate around the world without charge.

There are some marvelous software programs that allow for in-depth study of the Bible. One can search biblical texts and have several Bible commentaries at one's fingertips to better understand the meaning of the text. The amount and quality of Christian material available on the computer and over the internet is growing rapidly. It's a tool for spiritual growth all seniors ought to consider using.

Each year brings new developments in computer technology that expands these capabilities. There are countless opportunities for seniors to have mental activity that is healthy and will help them grow in knowledge and understanding, if they will learn to use the computer. Most areas of the country provide free classes to help seniors use the computer, if not a local community college will have a low cost class and most public libraries will have computers that can be used free of charge.

The computer is critical for learning, communication, and mental growth, so don't pass it by. Computers are easy to learn to use and they open up a whole new world.

Many seniors can get routine mental activity through playing games regularly like chess, checkers, scrabble, or bridge. Others do crossword, Sudoku, or other puzzles. It is important that seniors routinely and systematically involve themselves in activities that cause them to think and use their brain. As this is being written, some preliminary research results have been released which indicate that seniors who are mentally active tend to have fewer incidents of

Alzheimer's disease. The brain it seems doesn't wear out, and if it's not diseased in some way, it continues to function well until death.

Dr. Gene Cohen M.D. has published a book recently entitled *The Mature Mind – The Positive Power of the Aging Brain.*[5] Dr. Cohen states that research regarding the aging brain proves that some older myths about the senior brain are false. In fact on page 4 he states the following about the aging brain:

1. The aging brain is continually re-sculpting itself in response to new learning and experience.
2. New brain cells form throughout life.
3. The brains emotional circuitry matures and becomes more balanced with age.
4. The brain's two hemispheres are more equally used by older adults.

Dr. Cohen essentially demonstrates that the older brain can be even better than the younger brain. As we age, we tend to develop what Cohen calls "developmental wisdom" which helps us adjust to life. We do tend to have our short term memory issues giving rise to the oft used term "senior moments" but there are the compensating factors that make the mature mind a wonderful and useful element of God's creation. Besides the "senior moments" give us some wonderful jokes and humor to laugh at.

---

[5] Gene D. Cohen, M.D. *The Mature Mind – The Positive Power of the Aging Brain* (New York, NY: Basic Books, 2006).

For seniors looking for some exciting activities and to get some planning help on what to do in their retirement years there is an internet web site that can be very helpful. An organization called Career Ventures has received foundation support to develop information and opportunities for "Baby Boomers" who want to use their retirement years productively. Their web site is www.civicventures.com. This is not a Christian organization per se but they have a wealth of information including that relating to Christian volunteer opportunities. By the way, if you would like information from this web site or the ones below, and you don't have a computer or internet connection, ask a friend who does. Maybe your grandchildren will help you with this. Just take the web addresses you want to check and sit with them and review the information. Civic Ventures includes information on work as well as volunteer opportunities.

Some seniors will of necessity or desire continue to work full or part-time. It is becoming more common for seniors to do this both because of the need for them in the economy and because inflation or stock market performance has diminished the retirement benefits they were counting on. Many companies and industries are now receptive to having seniors split or share a job so that two seniors in effect do the work of one fulltime employee. This is beneficial for the company as well as for the seniors. The company gets a job filled by two good workers who can cover for each other and who do not need health benefits, an increasing cost for companies. The seniors can earn some money and have time to do the things they like as well – it's a win-win situation.

For seniors, who need or want to work, a web site of interest is www.encorecareers.com. Here you can explore part and full-time work possibilities. This site also provides links to other helpful web sites.

The largest field of activity for Christian seniors is in volunteering to help others. Here seniors follow scriptural directions to use their gifts to help others. The joy and benefits from this type of activity are enormous. Many seniors will volunteer at their church, local school, or mission/food bank in their area, however, there are now Christian organizations that provide information about worldwide volunteer opportunities. One organization designed to help Christian seniors find volunteer opportunities can be found at the web site www.christianvolunteering.org. Here you can find volunteer opportunities of a wide variety and in countries all over the world. For seniors with recreational vehicles (RVs) there are some special organizations that have grown up to organize special volunteer opportunities for those who travel and vacation in RVs. Here are some web sites specializing in opportunities for them: www.sowerministry.org, the Missionary Assistance Program at www.mmap.org, and the Roving Volunteers at www.rvics.com.

Another activity seniors enjoy is travel. Many for the first time have the money and time to travel to places they have always wanted to go. There are numerous travel services around the country that will help book trips and tours for any place you might want to go. One organization dedicated to senior travel and learning is Elderhostel. They have programs all over the world including their own Elderhostel floating university. One can get on their mailing list by calling 1-800 454-5768. Their web site is www.elderhostel.org.

Many community colleges around the country offer courses for seniors at no or reduced costs. Most school districts in the country also have continuing education programs offering a wide variety of learning opportunities. Many four year colleges also offer lifelong learning programs. Many of these programs are open to anyone who wishes to attend. One does not have to be an alumnus in most cases. Just call your local college and ask if they have a lifelong learning program for seniors.

In summary there are more opportunities for seniors to be active than ever before and there is something for everyone. There is absolutely no excuse for any senior to become sedentary or lack opportunities for physical, mental, social, or spiritual exercise. There are countless chances to serve God and others and to grow in faith at the same time. Loneliness, boredom, and helplessness, those plagues of old age, can't possibly infect the Christian, if we just follow God's word and direction. We will "bear fruit in old age." Now let us look at our health and how best to stay "fresh and green."

Chapter 7 - Health –
Don't Leave Home Without It

It is Better to Use
Exercise to Preserve
Health than Medicine
To get it Back

I f we are to bear fruit in old age then we are going have to be healthy. Fortunately through science we are learning more all the time about what it takes to attain and stay hale and hearty. Interestingly much of what science is uncovering about how to stay fit is simply reinforcing what the Bible already says. The Bible tells us to live righteous lives, to treat our bodies as "Temples of the Holy Spirit," to serve others, and to avoid laziness, gluttony, and immorality. Let's look at what modern science is telling us about staying healthy.

In our earlier book on retirement, *Every Day Is Saturday*, my wife and I reproduced a list from the National Institute on Aging (a unit of the National Institutes of Health in Washington D.C.), which listed 10 things you should do if you want to live a healthy life in your senior years. They are:

1. Eat a balanced diet, including five helpings of fruits and vegetables each day.

2. Exercise regularly.

3. Get regular health checkups.

4. Don't smoke.

5. Practice safety habits at home to prevent falls and fractures and always wear your safety belt when driving.

6. Stay in contact with family and friends. Stay active through work, play, and community.

7. Avoid over exposure to sun and cold.

8. If you drink, moderation is the key. When you drink let someone else drive.

9. Keep personal and financial records in order to simplify budgeting and investing. Plan long term housing and money needs.

10. Keep a positive attitude toward life. Do things that make you happy.

Now all of these things are good suggestions but the list lacks the most important one. We would add a number 11.

11. Live your faith with vigor. Study God's word regularly, worship often, pray, enjoy regular fellowship with your brothers and sisters in Christ, and ask the Holy Spirit to guide you in new ways to use your gifts to help others and to share your faith and love with them. That's the staying righteous part the Bible emphasizes.

Let me expand on these and some other matters that will lead to health in our senior years.

Eating and Weight

One of the great dangers for seniors, particularly for those who do not exercise regularly is the accumulation of unwanted weight. As was mentioned earlier, a recent study released by the U.S. Government, Older Americans 2008; Key Indicators of Well-Being, states that 31% of those over 65 are obese. The study also indicates that 50% of the leisure time of seniors is spent watching TV. Watching TV and eating is producing a major health problem in the USA. Obesity is linked to numerous health problems including heart and cardiovascular diseases, diabetes, osteoarthritis, some cancers, and sleep apnea among others.

One can see how America's health problems will be compounded if our seniors don't live healthier life styles. With an increasing senior population of Baby Boomers coming we are asking for a health system breakdown if over 30% of our seniors are obese and have even a portion of the health problems associated with it.

For Christians being overweight or obese is not only a potential health problem but it may also be a sin and a condition that restricts activity and shortens life. The Bible has several statements condemning gluttony and drunkenness. In one in Proverbs 23:20-21 we read, *"Do not join those who drink too much wine or gorge themselves on meat, for drunkards and gluttons become poor and drowsiness clothes them in rags."* Those seniors who want to stay "fresh and Green" will not over indulge and they will work to keep themselves in good physical shape.

It is important to eat a balanced diet and to avoid over eating in our senior years. We tend to need fewer calories as we age and of necessity we will probably get less exercise. As one who loves to eat and enjoys food, I have found that if I chew my food longer I enjoy it just as much but I eat a good deal less. A recent study suggested that if a person chewed their food longer they could save 70 calories a meal on average. I don't know about that, but I do know it works for me and on a regular basis I now look for senior menus at restaurants, which have smaller portions and save money. I now have no hesitancy to ask for a box to take uneaten food home for a second meal. I now simply eat less and enjoy it more. A good rule is to eat half as much and chew twice as long. You get just as much enjoyment from eating on half the calories.

As mentioned earlier, I have been using the term obese as defined by the U.S. Government standards. The National Institutes of Health (NIH) and the American Health Foundation have developed a standard that we can all use to determine if we are underweight, normal weight, overweight, obese, or gross obese. The standard is called the Body Mass Index (BMI). It is figured using the following formulas:

Weight Factor = 703 x (weight in pounds)
Height Factor = $(\text{height in inches})^2$
Body Mass Index (BMI) =   Weight Factor / Height Factor

For example, if a person weighed 175 pounds and was 5 feet 10 inches tall (70"), the computations would look like this:

Weight Factor = 703 x 175 = 123075

Height Factor = 70^2 = 4900

BMI = 123075 / 4900 = 25.107

We can then apply BMI numbers against the Body Mass Index scores that have been developed by the U.S. Government as follows:

Body Mass Index

0 – 18.5   Underweight

18.6 – 24.9   Normal weight range

25 – 29.9   Overweight (Increased Health Risks)

30 - 40   Obese (Definite Health Risks)

40+   Gross Obesity (Serious Health Risks)

Given the example above the person's BMI is at the top of the normal range with no real health risks. The person is, however, where, if they begin to gain weight, their health risks would begin to gradually increase.

Obviously it is difficult for one index to take everything in a person's individual situation into account and the BMI isn't a precision tool. However, the BMI has been well researched and is valid as a measurement for calculating our health risks. Anyone who is close to

30 or over on the BMI should consult a physician because of their significantly increased health risk.

Exercise

I know of no single prescription for health mentioned more than exercise. As we mentioned earlier, the human body was intended to be used. The body has built in maintenance systems that only work effectively if the body is used and the blood is pumping. A recent study showed that health is significantly improved if people even take a walk three times a week for 30 minutes each time. There isn't anyone who can't find the time to do this.

The more a person exercises regularly the better their physical condition is likely to be and the healthier they will become. For many people exercise is boring and uncomfortable and therefore they avoid it. The key to success is to make exercise fun. This can be done in many ways. Exercising with a friend, walking in a mall, setting goals, watching TV, listening to good music or talk radio, or reading while exercising are just some ways people make exercise more palatable. And if you exercise regularly reward yourself by doing something you particularly enjoy when you finish.

Walking is arguably the best exercise and something nearly everyone can do. Even in the winter in cold areas, malls and some mega churches have inside walking areas where you can walk distances even in bad weather. For those who wish to get in the best of physical condition a balanced exercise program should be developed that combines using weights and working out all the major muscle groups as well as combining a walking or jogging program. I personally work out three times a week for one and a half hours each time with weights and floor exercises, and on the days in between I walk for 30 to 40 minutes. This exercise program allows me to eat almost anything I want without gaining weight and it helps keep me in good physical shape with a BMI about 25. In short, I am investing only about 6 hours a week to maintain a good level of physical conditioning. Exercise is a great investment in ones health and longevity. Being in good physical shape also contributes to ones mental and spiritual health.

One caveat needs to be made here. If a person does not have a regular exercise program, and they are overweight, an exercise program should not be started unless they have had a physical and received a doctor's OK to begin. In most cases a person should start such a program slowly and gradually build it up to the desired level.

It is also a good health practice to have an annual physical as a preventive measure. Most progressive health insurance plans now provide for such a doctor's visit realizing that if things are caught early they can usually be cured quickly and at less cost. Preventive medicine works and has the potential for saving our national healthcare system a lot of money.

Obviously those who like active sports like tennis, golf, volleyball, swimming, running, basketball, bowling, softball etc. have a built in advantage with exercise built into an activity they already enjoy.

The last decade or two has seen the rapid development of organized senior sports including the Senior Olympics. There are organized leagues in many metropolitan areas for seniors in many sports so competition can be enjoyed well into the senior years. In Appendix A the reader will find web sites they can go to get information about senior sports in their area.

Accidents

Studies show that accidents, particularly falls, cause serious health problems for seniors. One study frequently quoted indicates that roughly 30% of seniors 65 and over have a fall every year. As we age our muscles and sense of balance may decline somewhat and we become more likely to fall. By the way, one of the great advantages of an exercise program is that a senior's good conditioning makes falling less likely, and if you fall you are less likely to be injured.

Particularly damaging to seniors are falls where a hip is broken. Fortunately today we have hip replacements and even a very bad hip fracture can often be repaired or replaced with the person back on their feet in a relatively short period of time. Hip fractures, however, are serious, can lead to long periods of inactivity, and even death.

Always wearing seat belts in the car can save many seniors serious injuries. Wearing seat belts is an important factor in adding to longevity.

What Not To Do

Seniors should not smoke or become over reliant on drugs to sleep or calm their nerves. A strong faith ought to make these less necessary. The "peace that passes understanding" which God gives his people is the best sleeping medication available.

Some studies seem to show that drinking alcoholic beverages in moderation particularly red wine can actually promote health. Moderation here is defined as no more than one or two drinks per day. Some Christians believe that total abstinence is the only biblically approved position to take. It is hard to make the case for total abstinence from scripture; however, the case for avoiding drunkenness is clear and persuasive. Avoiding all alcohol is certainly the safest course for the Christian, but drinking in moderation is not a sin and it can add a pleasurable dimension to the lives of those who enjoy it.

Avoiding over exposure to the sun can also help a senior avoid problems particularly skin cancers. This doesn't mean avoid the sun it means avoid over exposure to the sun. We need some sun because the sun's rays produce vitamin D and have a health benefit. Over exposure would be lying out in a hot sun for over 20 minutes without a highly rated sunscreen on. The older we get the more we need to take care here. It doesn't mean we can't go to the beach or have a good time swimming, but it does mean if we are going to have an extended time in the sun we need to put on a sun screen with a Sun Protection Factor (SPF) rating of 30 or higher - and generally the higher the SPF rating the better.

Becoming a "Couch Potato" is perhaps the most harmful thing a senior can do. Watching TV develops the inactivity mentioned earlier that impels one toward being overweight. The lack of exercise and a tendency to snack while watching can be damaging. If one is watching TV for a period of time, you should get up periodically walk around and stretch. Your body will love you for it. You might also do some hand, arm, and leg exercises periodically to break the spell of inactivity. If you are working for long periods on the computer, take some planned breaks and walk around a bit to give the mind a break and the body a short work out, both will benefit and love you for it.

What You Should Do

Staying active physically, mentally, and spiritually are the best things to do. There is recent scientific evidence that seems to indicate that people who are mentally active tend to have less Alzheimer's disease. There are many things seniors can do to stay mentally alert including doing crossword puzzles, Sudoku puzzles, playing scrabble, playing card games and becoming involved in various lifelong learning programs offered by most colleges and school districts around the country. Traveling and learning make a good combination as does engaging in a formal program of Bible study. Reading can also exercise our minds. As was mentioned earlier, we can learn until the day we die. The healthy mind can continue to make new neural connections as long as we are alive.

In my book, *Does God Laugh?,* I have a section where I discuss some fascinating research that has developed in recent years regarding a bodily secretion called an endorphin. Endorphin, which means morphine within, is a secretion from the anterior portion of our pituitary gland and it has amazing properties. Endorphins relieve pain, strengthen our immune systems and help us fight disease, increase longevity, and promote a general sense of well being. They are a kind of miracle drug secreted by the body under certain conditions.

Scientists have found that the conditions which promote the secretion of endorphins are listening to good music, laughing, exercise, and hugging and making love. In short, we can promote good health and healing, add to our happiness, and extend our lives if we engage in these activities on a regular basis.

In writing my book on laughter I researched a group of comedians that were born around the turn of the 20th century. They were comedians with whom I grew up. There were about 15 of them and included Bob Hope, George Burns, Milton Berle, Groucho Marx, Fibber McGee and Molly, Red Skelton, Jack Benny, Lucille Ball, and others. When these comedians were born in the late 1800s and early 1900s the life expectancy was 47 years. When I calculated the average age at death of this group of comedians I found it was 77. They had outlived their peers by an average of 30 years. What caused this? One factor may have been that they made their living by laughing. Some also added music to their acts. This scientific evidence seems again to just confirm a biblical principle stated in Proverbs 17:22 where we read, "*A cheerful heart is a good medicine, but a crushed spirit dries up the bones.*"

The medical community in America now recognizes the roll that humor can play in healing. Some hospitals actually have humor carts in their children's wards because they recognize that if children are laughing they are also healing.

Some will also remember the popular movie *Patch Adams* starring Robin Williams. The main character was Dr. Hunter Adams who spent his life trying to convince his medical colleagues that humor can assist healing. Dr. Adams founded the Gesundheit Institute in West Virginia which is dedicated to promoting healing through humor. There is now a professional organization called the American Association for Therapeutic Humor (AATH) which is also dedicated to this proposition. In short, humor is good for us and looking for opportunities to laugh can add to our longevity, as the Bible indicates.

Another interesting study I saw in the paper recently showed a correlation between dental flossing and longevity. Evidently keeping a clean healthy mouth with healthy gums, and few if any cavities, is a positive factor in improving health and extending life. This makes sense since the mouth is at the beginning of the digestive system and if the entrance to the system is healthy the rest of the system will be at less risk for disease.

In summary, if seniors want to have a healthy, happy, and productive last 1/3 of life they can certainly have it, if there are some things they avoid and some things they do. Following what I call the four Ls isn't a bad way to remember what we can do. We can have a great life if we will love, laugh, learn, and listen. Those things plus staying active, serving God, and helping others guarantees we will stay "fresh and green" and "bear fruit in old age."

Chapter 8 - Money - Use It Wisely,
Don't Let It Use You

Give all you can because
No one ever saw
A Hearse Pulling a U-Haul

T he Bible says in I Timothy 6:10 that *"The love of money is the root of all kinds of evil."* That is certainly true, but we can deal with money without falling in love with it or having it consume our lives. Note the Bible says it is the love of money not the possession of it that is the root of sin. Money is a necessary commodity that helps us achieve our goals, but it should be a *means to an end not an end in itself.*

Dealing effectively with finances is becoming more important for the senior simply because we are living longer and we need to stretch our retirement income over a much longer period than in the past. We can no longer depend entirely on Social Security (SS) to take care of our financial needs until we leave this world. Most seniors will have saved for retirement and should have enough income from (SS), a 401k plan, a pension plan, and/or annuities to be financially secure.

Hopefully most seniors will have adequately prepared for retirement so they can turn their lives to fulltime Christian service and fellowship. Unfortunately a study reported recently by the *Consumer*

Bankruptcy Project[6] indicates that bankruptcies for older Americans are going up significantly. During the period of the study (1991-2007) bankruptcies for those aged 55-64 were up 40%, for those 65-74 they were up 125%, and for those 75-84 they were up an incredible 433%. The rapid increases point to the importance of managing our resources wisely.

The traditional rule-of-thumb financial planners have used to help people plan for retirement is that people will need 70% of their pre-retirement income to maintain the same living standard in retirement as before. This will vary some by income level but it is still a reasonable rule-of-thumb. Seniors will find some expenses for food, clothing, housing, and 401k contributions go down but healthcare, travel, and entertainment expenses may increase. It is important when approaching retirement to develop a realistic budget for living to insure you will be able to live comfortably. It's always safe to over-estimate expenses and to under-estimate income a bit.

Planning finances for the last 1/3 of life is complicated by the fact that some expenses and financial conditions can't be easily projected and yet will inevitably change. For example one area where expenses for seniors often go up is the area of healthcare and drugs. Inflation is another factor we can't easily project. If a senior has good health insurance and Medicare, they are largely protected except from the most catastrophic situations. The cost-of-living increases in Social

---

[6] The Consumer Bankruptcy Project was reported on Newsmax.com, August 27, 2008, and examined bankruptcies filed between 1991 and 2007.

Security and most pension plans help, but they often understate true inflation and do not entirely compensate for increased living costs. The Federal Cost of Living Adjustment, according to many economists, actually under states the true cost of living that impacts most people. In short, it is essential for most seniors to plan their finances carefully and to err in the direction of over stating their needs and the inflation that is inevitable.

Here are some basic attitudes and principles that are important and helpful in managing the financial resources God has given us:

It all belongs to God. The Christian's attitude toward money and worldly possessions is that we simply hold all things in trust for God. This attitude should prevail in retirement as well. We can't take it with us though many of us will wish to leave some behind for our children or favorite charities. To carefully set, plan, and accomplish financial goals is important to our well being in the senior years. I'll say more about how to do this shortly.

Don't worry about money. "God will provide" is a valid principle at any stage of life and it is true for the senior Christian. This doesn't mean we shouldn't plan, budget, and practice being frugal. It means we shouldn't worry about it. Someone has said that happiness is somewhere between having too much and having too little. In the USA even our poor are rich by worldly standards. As we'll see, while we shouldn't worry about money, we should plan wisely in terms of how we use what God has given us.

Someone asked a wealthy man one day how much they needed to be considered rich. They were expecting a monetary figure but the answer they got was, "You are rich if you have a place to live, food to eat, and friends." Not a bad answer.

Plan and budget wisely. It is simply good stewardship to plan and budget. We need to use our resources wisely. Christians who follow biblical principles for the use of money are known for being humble, modest, and generous. Wasting money and resources on conspicuous consumption is simply not a Christian practice or something God will honor.

Save all you can, and give all you can. Jesus suggests in Matthew 6 that it is not wise for us to lay up treasures for ourselves here on earth but he suggests in Matthew 6:20, *"But lay up for yourselves treasures in heaven where moth and rust do not corrupt and where thieves do not break through and steal."* How do we make deposits in our heavenly bank account? We do it by giving to God's causes and by doing good works here on earth. Not only is it good to give to others it is more fulfilling and fun than spending the money on some frivolous self-centered item. And Christians should remember that *we can't out give God*. But as a friend of mine said, "It sure is fun trying."

Giving a tithe to God's work is a good place to start, if you're not already doing it, and an invitation to God to pour out blessings upon you as he promised in Malachi. In Malachi 3:10 we read, *"...and prove me herewith, saith the Lord of Hosts, if I will not open you the windows of heaven and pour out a blessing, that there shall not be room enough to receive it."* Giving a tithe is undoubtedly the most important thing we can do to insure our financial security both here and in the life to come.

Get out of debit and use credit cautiously. The Bible has many things to tell us about how to view and use our money and one of them is in Proverbs where we are warned about debt. We read in Proverbs 22:7, *"The borrower is slave to the lender."* Financial institutions make it easy to borrow money because that's how they make money. We need to resist the ease with which we can be lured into debt and avoid the circumstances that are driving record numbers of Americans and seniors into bankruptcy. There are very few circumstances where Christians should accumulate any debt that can't be paid off in full at the end of each month. Buying a home or possibly a car may be the major ones. Getting debt free and staying that way is certainly the best course for Christians.

Set goals. Set annual goals for spending and for monitoring your net worth. Net worth is a broad financial measure that tracks all your personal assets and liabilities and allows one the opportunity to track on a global basis how they are doing from year to year. In Appendix E I have provided some forms easily used to budget and calculate net worth.

At least once a year, usually at year's end, every Christian or family should compute their net worth in order to check their progress from year to year. This is in the financial area the equivalent of taking an annual physical in the health area.

Seek good advice. If you are not an expert in the financial area, seek good Christian advice. Often churches have people in them who will gladly counsel people on financial matters and hopefully all churches provide a class or workshop for their members on what the Bible has to say about handling money. If you want a high level of professional assistance, you may want to pay for the services of a financial planner. If you do this make sure the person is well trained and has either a CFP (Certified Financial Planner) or a ChFC after their names. This insures they have had specialized training and have passed a comprehensive exam. They should also be certified by the Securities and Exchange Commission of the U.S. Government. If you would like to find such a person in your area, you can go to the web site of their professional association the Financial Planning Association (FPA) at www.fpanet.org. Certified Public Accountants (CPA) also do this work but make sure they have a PFS (Personal Financial Specialist) certification.

Dave Ramsay is a wonderful Christian financial advisor with a national radio program and several books. His advice is sound and any of his workshops, seminars, or courses are well worth taking. I have also found that Money Magazine is worth taking. Their financial advice is comprehensive and wise, though it is not necessarily offered from the Christian perspective.

We'll talk more about this later but you might also need an attorney to handle financial matters related to your estate, taxes, and will. If so, seek one who is a Christian and one who specializes in estate planning, wills, and trusts.

Invest wisely. If you are blessed with excess resources invest them wisely. You may want to use a financial planner or investment adviser to do this. Be advised, however, that there are those who will provide these services free of charge. Not much in life is free and one must use these services, if you do, with care. Banks, insurance companies, mutual fund companies, brokerages, and comprehensive financial institutions will often offer free financial planning services, however, each one has an agenda, and while they may be very ethical, they make their money from selling you financial products like annuities, mutual funds, insurance policies, and stocks. Their advice may be good but always double check their advice with some objective third party you trust and be aware these organizations are in business to make a profit off selling you products and services.

Generally speaking as one gets older they should become more conservative in their investments because if you lose capital in an investment there is not a lot of time to make it up and replace it. Diversity is an element of being more conservative. Generally speaking, the more diverse one's investments are, the less risk is involved. Seniors should take care to have a diversity of investments. Below are some categories of investments and their risk levels. As indicated, generally as one ages they should have more investments in the low and medium risk categories. The percentage in the high risk area should be very low and at a point where if it were all lost overnight it wouldn't impact ones living standard in any way.

Low Risk

Certificates of Deposit

Treasury Bills and Bonds

Money Market Funds (MFs)

Savings Bonds

Tax-deferred Annuities

Savings Accounts

Medium Risk

Income Stocks

Utility Stocks

Real Estate Investment Trusts (REITs)

Blue Chip Corporate Stocks and Mutual Funds

High Quality (AAA, and AA rated) Corporate Bonds

Tax Free Municipal Bonds

Balanced Mutual Funds (diversified portfolios)

Gold, Silver, and Precious Metals Stocks and Mutual Funds

High Risk

Growth Stocks

Low rated and Junk Bonds (BBB rated and below)

Small Cap and Growth Mutual Funds

Penny Stocks and Mutual Funds

Collectibles

Some financial planners would recommend a mixture of investments based upon your age:

	Ages 50-65	Ages 65-75	Ages 75+
Low Risk Investments	40%	50%	65%
Medium Risk Investments	30%	30%	25%
High Risk Investments	30%	20%	10%

Obviously there is a risk/reward ratio at work in the investment world meaning the higher the risks one takes the greater are the possible returns and the possibility of principle loss. The lower the risk is the lower the returns generally, and the lower the possibility of loss.

These are just rough rules-of-thumb and individual situations will differ widely, therefore, special advice should be applied to each situation.

If you need more money. Some seniors may find their retirement income is beginning to fall short. If this happens there are some ways this situation can be handled. They are:

1. **Go back to work or continue working**. If you see the financial need coming before you retire keep working. Many companies are grateful to have faithful employees continue full-time or part-time. Some companies will split jobs so two employees do one job but each only works half time – it is called job sharing. There are many

companies who seek to employ seniors part-time because generally their work habits, trustfulness, and integrity are high plus they do not need healthcare, which is one of the companies highest employee related costs. Seniors are prized for their knowledge and experience, so if you need extra cash opportunities are available. Go to your local American Association of Retired Persons (AARP) and inquire about programs for seniors and a list of employers who are senior friendly. Home Depot, for example, has a program with AARP to train and use seniors in their stores.

2. **Start a business**. Many seniors find pleasure and money in starting a small business. Often a hobby can be turned into a money making proposition. Woodworking, painting, photography, catering, sowing, knitting, or a hundred other endeavors can be turned into full or part-time businesses. We all remember Colonel Sanders who started Kentucky Fried Chicken after he retired. Even if income isn't the primary focus, many of these endeavors can meet many of the other needs a senior has. One caveat here, however, if you are over 65 and receiving Social Security if you make over a certain amount you will forfeit some of your Social Security check. You can find out what this amount is currently by calling 1-800-772-1213 or going to the SS web site at: www.ssa.gov.

3. **Do a reverse mortgage**. A fairly recent financial instrument is the reverse mortgage. In this transaction a bank or other financial institution actually buys your home from you and pays a monthly

fee to you for life based on the value of your home and life expectancy. Be advised, however, that these transactions can be expensive. They should be carefully examined and all the fine print scrutinized before going ahead with such an action. In these reverse mortgages, upon your death the home goes to the financial institution and does not become a part of your estate, which could be left to heirs. These mortgages work best if income must be increased and if leaving a home to your children or heirs isn't an issue. The National Center for Home Equity Conversion (NCHEC) is a nonprofit association that provides help in this area. You may visit their web site at www.reverse.org.

4. **Use your home equity for income**. If you have a great deal of equity in your home, you can borrow that through a home equity loan to meet expenses or to invest. When you borrow, however, there is a cost and the loan must be paid back, so all of this must be calculated in the equation to determine if this is a good way to go. Another way to use home equity is to sell your home, move into something smaller, and take the difference in price and invest it or buy an annuity that will pay a regular income for life. You must be careful in making these transactions and insure that they are done correctly, in good order, and in your best interests. A good financial adviser can be very helpful in considering these options and can often save you more than their cost.

5. **Cash in life insurance policies**. Life insurance isn't as important for a senior as it was earlier in life when there were dependants.

Many life insurance policies have a cash value and/or might be convertible into an annuity that could pay a monthly income for life. Check your life insurance policies for possible options. In some cases seniors might better take the cash value of the policy and invest it in a mutual fund for later use, if needed.

Prudent financial planning is what God wants us to do. He expects us to use our resources wisely and in accordance with his teaching. As someone once said, "He who dies with the most toys is still dead." Using money wisely and prudently is God's desire for us. We should use it not let it use us, as it does for so many who come to love money more than anything else. If we use our money here as God directs us, we will not only meet God later but we'll also meet our money again in our heavenly bank account.

Now let's look at that wonderful transition we will have as we return one day to the home office.

Chapter 9 - Death
The Christian's Return to the Home Office

Christ is Risen and
You O' Death
Are Annihilated
- John Chrysostom

Billy Graham once suggested that too many Christians avoid thinking about death because they think it is an unpleasant subject when it is not. Certainly it shouldn't be for the Christian. The fear of death is Satan's weapon against us. In Philippians 1:21 we read, *"For to me, to live is Christ and to die is gain."*

I believe it is important to discuss death because the fear of death in too many cases inhibits seniors, stifles activity, and steals the joy of living in the golden years. Unless we come to grips with our own deaths we can't possibly enjoy and be productive in what can be our most fruitful years. Too many seniors, even Christians, allow worry about death and dying to rob their latter years of much of the joy that could be theirs. So let's review what we know about death.

The Bible tends to refer to death as falling asleep or of passing through a door, gate, or curtain. It is, in effect, a quick passage from this world to the next. For the Christian it is a passage from this world into the presence of God. In I Corinthians 15:54-57 we read, *"...death is swallowed up in victory. O death where is your sting? O grave where is thy victory? The sting of death is sin ... But thanks be to God which giveth us the victory through our Lord Jesus Christ."* For the Christian the sting is gone and the victory is assured.

Most, if not all Christians, I believe, are not as concerned about death as they are about the possible pain and distress that might accompany their getting there. I will address pain a bit later, but there is good news about how medical science is conquering pain. Before addressing pain let me address what we know about death and what happens when we go through that door or curtain.

I believe, though some Christians will doubt it, that God has given us a glimpse of what is beyond through the experiences some folks have had with what are called near-death experiences (NDE) or a pre-death experiences (PDE). Thousands of people have had these experiences and an extensive literature has grown up around the subject.

Dr. Raymond Moody and Betty Eadie are two authors who have written extensively on the subject of NDEs and PDEs, each writing several books on the subjects. The most popular recent Christian author to write on the subject is Don Piper whose book *90 Minutes in Heaven*[7] hit the best seller list. Don had a horrific auto accident and was pronounced dead. He reported an amazing account of spending 90 minutes in heaven. Don's account of what he saw and heard bears similarities to what the Apostle John saw as revealed in Revelations Chapter 4.

---

[7] Don Piper, *90 Minutes in Heaven.* (Grand Rapids, Michigan, Revell: 2004).

My wife and I spent some time reviewing the PDE and NDE material in preparation for writing our book *Seven for Heaven.* In this book we interviewed Christian hospice patients as they were dying. We wondered whether we would find that any of these people would have a PDE or NDE. We concluded that three of them did have such experiences. A long time hospice nurse told us she had experienced numerous PDEs, and in fact, she was so convinced they were real that she had instructed her family that on her death bed they were under no conditions to allow doctors to medicate her because she wanted to experience the PDE fully without any drug interference.

As mentioned earlier, some Christians believe PDEs and NDEs have connections to some of the New Aged religious phenomenon and therefore reject them. I can only say that no less a Christian than Billy Graham believes in PDEs since he was there when his grandmother experienced one before she died. Graham tells about it in his book *Hopes for the Troubled Soul.*[8] As she was dying Billy said his grandmother looked up and said she saw Jesus and her deceased husband Ben. She further noted that Ben had his leg and eye back. Ben had lost them both in a Civil War battle. After reporting this to those around her bed she died peacefully. Was it real or a mind playing tricks on her? I think it was real and that there is a mountain of evidence to substantiate that such things occur.

---

[8] Billy Graham, *Hopes for the Troubled Soul.* (Dallas, Texas: Word Publishing Co., 1991).

There are some common denominators for people who have had NDEs which I think are interesting:

1. They go through a dark tunnel.
2. They have feelings of peace and quiet.
3. They have a "out of body" experience where they often view their bodies from the outside.
4. They see a being of "light" sometimes reported to be Jesus.
5. They report being surrounded by a light, which feels like a strong love. While the light is strong it does not hurt their eyes.
6. They report meeting others, often friends and relatives who have died.
7. They report returning to their bodies, often unhappy at having to leave the "light."

The only negative NDEs are reported by those who have attempted suicide or were atheists. They reported hell-like experiences.

Dr. Raymond Moody, a medical doctor, after studying numerous cases of NDEs, says in his book *The Light Beyond*[9] that people who have had these experiences have some marvelous outcomes. As a result of their experiences they:

1. No longer fear dying.
2. Have a new sense of the importance of love.
3. Feel a new sense of connection with all things.
4. Have a new appreciation for learning.

---

[9] Raymond Moody, *The Light Beyond*. (New York: Bantam Books, 1998).

5. Develop a new feeling of control.

6. Feel a new sense of urgency about life.

7. Have a better developed spiritual side.

8. Experience difficulty reentering the "real" world.

Now, I would ask, if thousands of people have experienced these NDEs and have nearly unanimously had the above reactions, particularly #1, how can Christians ever again fear what lies beyond?

I believe, in spite of what some critics say, that God has through these NDEs and PDEs given us a glimpse of what lies beyond, and it is wonderful beyond belief. I have heard Don Piper try to describe the music he heard and the colors he saw in his 90 minutes in heaven and his description goes beyond anything we have ever heard or imagined. It's consistent with what the Bible says about it. I personally can't wait.

The bottom line is that no Christian should ever have one fearful moment worrying about what happens when we die. There is the process of getting there, however, and many Christians are rightly concerned about possible pain and circumstances of dying.

My wife has been a volunteer for years with the hospice movement serving as a volunteer working with the dying and their families. We were concerned when we wrote our book *Seven for Heaven* about the pain levels the dying might be suffering. We came away from our experience much impressed with what medical science has accomplished in dealing with pain. While all of our subjects were dying of disease, primarily cancer, we found that the hospice program did a wonderful job of controlling the pain. Not one of our patients died grimacing in pain and only one had suffered seriously.

Medical science now trains and certifies doctors in the treatment of pain. Science has developed numerous drugs and techniques to deal with the wide variety and types of pains. The key to dealing with a painful illness is to make sure you have a doctor specifically trained to deal with pain and then do your best to communicate to the doctor where the pain is and what type of pain it is. With that information doctors can relieve or seriously mitigate any pain you might encounter. To me personally finding this out was a great comfort because it was the pain, not the dying, which has concerned me most, as I advance toward the wonderful day I'll meet my maker.

By the way, while this chapter is being written the newspaper has reported that scientists have developed a new pain killer which is 30 times more potent than morphine. Until now morphine has been arguably the most used pain killer of last resorts. We can expect that modern science will continue to work to alleviate pain and will continue to produce new procedures and drugs to combat one of our greatest threats.

While I do not personally believe in euthanasia, I do believe it is correct to sedate and medicate patients who are suffering even at the risk of shortening life. This is also the position of the Roman Catholic Church which has studied and spoken out on the issue.

In the Catechism of the Catholic Church we read the following:

"Even if death is thought imminent, the ordinary care owed to a sick person cannot be legitimately interrupted. The use of pain killers to alleviate the sufferings of the dying, even at the risk of shortening their days, can be morally in conformity with human dignity if death is not willed as either an end or a means, but only foreseen and tolerated as inevitable."[10]

In short, I believe the Catholic Church has it exactly right on this matter and the policy should be a comfort to any who may face a debilitating and painful illness.

Interestingly the legal position in the United States regarding physician assisted suicide and the right-to-die closely parallels the position of the Catholic Church. In 1997 the U.S. Supreme Court dealt with these issues in two cases, Washington v. Glucksburg and Quill v. Vacho. The court ruled that there was not an inherent right-to-die in the constitution, however, they stated that it was legal for a physician to give pain medications to a terminally ill patient in the form of opiates and barbiturates even if one of the outcomes might be to hasten death. So, doctors can even induce unconsciousness with drugs in a terminally ill patient in order to relieve pain, even if doing so hastens death. This again is basically the position of the Catholic Church.

At this writing two states have laws permitting physician assisted suicide. Oregon passed it in 1995 and Washington in 2008. Since the Oregon law was passed about 400 people have been assisted

---

[10] Catechism of the Catholic Church released in 1994 (subheading I, Euthanasia, 2279).

in suicide. Several legal challenges have been brought against the law but all have failed. In other states in the U.S. physician assisted suicide is illegal. So that is the current legal status at the moment.

If death to the Christian is a wonderful admission into the presence of God, a reunion with friends and relatives who have gone on before, and the beginning of a new everlasting life, what is there to fear or be anxious over? If modern science has largely defeated the pain of a lingering debilitating illness, what is there to fear? Death may still involve momentary stress from a heart attack or stroke but these conditions often quickly result in unconsciousness. Even in a serious accident where major injuries occur our bodies quickly shut down and we enter shock or unconsciousness and escape the consciousness of unbearable pain.

Some will fear death because it means a separation from friends, relatives, and perhaps a mate who will be left behind, however, the fact that the Christian has the true assurance of a reunion ought to help offset that plus the wonderful reunion with those who have gone before will be fantastic. They've been waiting for us.

Certainly life as we age will produce some aches and pains but nothing unbearable. What pain we do suffer can even serve a healthy purpose, if it reminds us and helps us appreciate just a bit about the anguish Jesus suffered on the cross for our sins. I was told not long ago about a devout lady who was dying and in severe pain. She refused the pain killing drugs that were offered to her because she said she wanted to experience just a bit of what Jesus went through to save us, so she could appreciate more what Jesus did for us. She died in pain, but she did it for a reason. The decision to die in pain was a personal one for her and certainly not required of us, but it does remind us that the pain we may suffer here is just a sample of what Jesus suffered, and it should increase our appreciation and understanding of what he did for us.

There is a wonderful organization that has developed to help people who are dying to do so with dignity and without pain. This organization is called hospice. Let me say a word about them here because they are a wonderful resource for people who are dying of a serious illness.

The word hospice comes from the Latin word *hospitum* meaning "guesthouse." It was originally used to describe a place of shelter for sick and weary travelers returning from religious pilgrimages. Hospice is both a contemporary and an ancient concept of care. Hospices have comforted critically ill and dying people, as well as their families, since at least the Middle Ages of European history. England is credited with founding the first twentieth-century hospice in 1905 – the St. Joseph's Hospice.

During the 1960s, Dr. Cicely Saunders, a British physician, began the modern hospice movement by establishing St. Christopher's Hospice near London. St. Christopher's organized a team approach to professional care for the dying and was the first program to use modern pain management techniques to care for the dying compassionately.

The first American hospice began providing care in 1974 in Connecticut. Literally hundreds of hospices have been organized all over the United States since then. Many are situated in hospitals, but others are designed as "free standing" units like St Joseph's and St. Christopher's, in England. Some hospices are affiliated with religious groups while others are public and non-sectarian. It is now fair to say that wherever one resides in the U.S.A. there is a hospice in the area that is available should their services be needed.

The hospice is a deliberate effort to meet the medical, social, religious, and psychological needs of the dying. The organization specializes in palliative care meaning that the patient's comfort is primary. This care even takes priority over curative care though the latter is not disregarded. The hospice movement maximizes the use of the latest techniques in pain management, which have grown rapidly in recent years.

While there are a growing number of hospice facilities around the country where people can go to die in a family friendly environment, roughly 70% of hospice patients choose to die at home. Hospice is a concept of care. It is one of the best examples of the holistic approach to health care delivery. Hospice is holistic because it not only takes into account the multiple dimensions of the patient's psychological and spiritual needs, it also incorporates supporting health professionals, family members, and friends in the caring procedure.

Today there are more than 3100 hospice programs in the United States. In 1998 hospice programs cared for 540,000 patients and this has increased significantly today.

If you or your family should be facing death from a serious illness or injury I would strongly urge you to consider contacting a nearby hospice program. Any physician or hospital can put one in contact with a hospice or you can find one by going to one of the organizations or web sites listed below.

The National Hospice and Palliative Care Organization

1700 Diagonal Drive (Suite 300)

Alexanderia, VA 22314

Phone: 1-703 873-1500

Informational Hotline: 1-800 658-8898

Web site: www.nhpco.org

Hospice Foundation of America

2001 S St. N.W. #300

Washington, D.C.

Phone: 1-800 854-3402

Web site: www.hospicefoundation.org

Now, in order for us to get rid of any apprehension about dying and to help us look forward even more to going home let's take a long look in the next chapter about what we will experience when we hit the tape and run right into the arms of Jesus and receive our crown.

Chapter 10 - Receiving Your Crown

Be Faithful Unto Death
And I Will Give You a
Crown of Life
– Revelations 2:10

Runners in a track meet always run to come in first and to get the medal or ribbon signifying that they won the race. This is on their minds as they practice and prepare and it motivates their efforts. They think about it constantly as do players on athletic teams who are motivated by winning the game or match. We Christians I believe need to spend more time thinking about the prize we will receive at the end of our individual life races. I believe we could and should think more about it in order to better understand and appreciate the efforts we need to make in order to receive our crowns. So what will our reward be for winning our races?

In the ancient Olympic Games the winners were given a crown woven from the branches of an olive tree. In the modern Olympic Games the winners receive gold metals. Second place finishers are given silver metals and third place finishers bronze metals. Those who finish the race of life and who "run thru the tape" receive a prize too. In Revelations 2:10 God says through the writing of the Apostle John, *"...Be faithful, even to the point of death, and I will give you the crown of life."* The Apostle Peter says that those who are faithful to the end will also be rewarded with a crown. We read in 1 Peter 5:4, *"And when the Chief Shepherd appears you will receive the crown of glory that will never fade away."* This promise is further reinforced in the book of James. We read there, James 1:12, *"Blessed is the man who perseveres under trial, because when he has stood the test, he will receive the crown of life that God has promised to those who love him."*

So what is this crown like? Will we wear it on our heads as the kings of old and the early Olympic champions did? Or does this crown of life or crown of glory have a deeper meaning? I think it's obviously the latter. This crown our God bestows on us when we run thru the tape is nothing less than eternal life with him in glory. So what will that be like? What is this prize we will actually receive as we break that tape? I think God has in various ways allowed us to get a glimpse of that experience. Let me see if I can paint a picture of what our crown, prize, or glory will be like.

I believe there are examples of the life beyond in the Bible, in contemporary life, and in the experiences of people who have had near-death experiences (NDEs) and pre-death experiences (PDEs). There are some amazing overlaps in all of these elements that I believe give us just a brief snapshot of what life may be beyond the finish line.

I would like to now try and paint a picture of what life will be like if we win the crown and get to spend eternity with God. The following descriptions come from a variety of sources that include scripture, books about PDEs and NDEs, from my wife and my experiences with dying hospice patients, and from the books of Randy

Alcorn[11] and Don Piper.[12] Randy Alcorn's book is by far the most complete book on the subject of heaven I have ever read. If the reader's interest in heaven is stimulated by what you read here I would urge you to get the Alcorn book to study the subject further.

Because the word picture developed below is a composite of many sources all mixed together I will not attempt to document each observation separately because each one may come from several sources. The word picture is solely mine based on what I have read, experienced, and found to be consistent with what I know about scripture.

When we "hit the tape" one of the first sensations we will experience is a light like no other light we have ever known. This light, which many people who have had near death experiences (NDEs) uniformly report, is exceptionally bright, but it doesn't hurt the eyes to look at it. The light also seems to have an emotional quality about it. The people who have experienced it say they felt loved like never before. In other words, the light conveyed a strong emotional feeling of being loved. Some NDEs saw this light emanating from a figure which many identified as being Jesus.

Light is an element that is consistently identified in the Bible as a characteristic of God and Jesus. In John 3:19 and John 1:1-9 Jesus is consistently referred to as light. The same is true in Matthew 4:6, and John 12:35. In 1 John 1:5 we read, *"...God is light; in him there is no*

---

[11] Randy Alcorn, *Heaven*, (Tyndale House Publishers: 2004).
[12] Don Piper, *90 Minutes in Heaven*, (Grand Rapids, Michigan: Revell, 2004).

darkness." In James 1:17 God is referred to as "*The Father of lights.*" In the Old Testament in the book of Habakkuk 1:4 we read about God, "*And his brightness was as light....*"

There are many instances in both New and Old Testaments where God appeared and in each case one of the characteristics of God's presence was a unique and over powering light. Moses experienced it on Mt. Sinai when he received the 10 Commandments (Exodus 34), the Apostle Paul was overcome by a light on the Damascus road (Acts 22:6-11), which Paul interpreted as the presence of God. Peter, James and John saw it on the mount where Jesus was transfigured described in Matthew 17:1-9 where we read, "*...there he was transfigured before them. His face shone like the sun, and his clothes became as a white light....*" There are other references in scripture to God as light; the concept is consistent, as is the converse namely references to Satan as the Prince of Darkness.

In Revelations the Apostle John is given a glimpse of Heaven and he writes in Revelation 22:5, "*There will be no more night. They will not need the light of a lamp or the light of the sun, for the Lord will give them light. And they will reign forever and ever.*"

Let me repeat that the experiences of the vast majority of NDEs is entirely consistent with the scriptural identification with God and light. This leads me to believe that the NDE experiences are real and just a brief glimpse of what is ahead for us.

So the case is powerfully made that once we cross the finish line we will be in an everlasting light never to know darkness again. This light which emanates from the presence of God will bath us in a feeling of love and peace that will last forever.

How can one not want to run thru that tape?

On the other side of the tape is a new body also. We seem to put on a new and unique body which has amazing properties. For example some NDEs reported that they had instant knowledge. Their minds essentially had the answers to questions as soon as their mind formed the question. Knowledge was direct and instantaneous. Some day we will know it all and we'll all know more than all the earthly Ph.D.s put together. We will also know everyone in heaven including our friends and relatives who have gone on before.

NDEs people report having relatives who have died coming to meet them. These folks are known and are perfect in their appearance. Any handicaps, blemishes, or age related hindrances are gone. People in heaven seem to all be perfect and reflective of an earthly age where they reached their prime. Billy Graham's grandmother saw her husband with Jesus before she died and her husband Ben had the leg and eye he'd lost in battle restored. Everyone in heaven will be perfect.

Our heavenly bodies will be like that of Jesus after his resurrection. You'll recall that Jesus appeared numerous times to his apostles and followers. In Luke 24:13-32 we read of Jesus meeting with two followers on the road to Emmaus. He talks with them and breaks bread with them. Only after instantaneously leaving them do they fully realize it was the risen Jesus with whom they had been walking and talking. In Matthew 28:8-18 Jesus appears to his followers at different times and it indicates they touched him and worshiped him. In Luke 24:36-44 Jesus suddenly appeared to the disciples in a closed room and invited them to touch his wounds from the crucifixion. Jesus also ate with his disciples. Jesus had a body that was fully physical, as ours are today, but it had other properties far beyond our bodies. He could appear and disappear instantaneously. Jesus was capable of what some call "thought travel." He wished to be somewhere and was instantly transported there through some amazing process.

Jesus' body passed through physical barriers as if they didn't exist. There were no physical hindrances to movement from one place to another.

It seems our resurrection bodies will have instant knowledge, thought travel capabilities, and the capability of enjoying eating and other pleasures. We'll be able to eat without getting fat or counting calories and the need for elimination will be gone. There'll be no need for "Johnny-on-the-spots" in heaven. We'll feel no pain only pleasure there. There'll be no need to sleep, we'll not get tired, and the work we do there will all be pure pleasure. The pain of work will be gone.

In Philippians 3:20 Paul reinforces all this where he states, "*But our citizenship is in heaven. And we eagerly await a savior from there, the Lord Jesus Christ, who ... will transform our lowly bodies so that they will be like his glorious body.*"

There will be music in heaven that is beyond our understanding. I've always thought that the Messiah, especially the Hallelujah Chorus, was God's sampling of what heaven's music would be like. Frederick Handel believed he was under God's influence when he composed the Messiah, and I believe he was. When King James of England first heard the Hallelujah Chorus he arose he was so moved. When the King stood up in those days everyone had to stand. That event has given rise to the custom often followed today that every time the Hallelujah Chorus is performed people arise for it. I believe this custom points us to the inspiration of this piece, but listen to what one visitor to heaven experienced.

Don Piper reports that in his 90 minutes in heaven he heard numerous pieces of music all playing at the same time. Many Hallelujah Choruses at the same time and instead of their being noise and a clashing of sounds he reported he heard each one separately and distinctly. Can you image that? Heavenly choruses, angelic choirs, all at the same time, and individually perceived, heard, and enjoyed. By the way, Don Piper's experience is similar to what is reported by John in Revelations 5:11 where we read, *"Then I looked and heard the voice of many angels, numbering thousands, and ten thousand times ten thousand. They encircled the throne and the living creatures and elders. In a loud voice they sang."*

What else will we experience? The presence of God will fill heaven and the Holy City. There will be everyone who has died in faith and we'll know and be known by everyone. There will be animals there including pets we had here on earth. Heaven will be a bit like the Garden of Eden before the fall but even better. The lions and lambs shall lie down together. Frankly the enormity of the magnificence of heaven is limited only by our human limitations in comprehending it. That's what is awaiting us when we "run thru the tape."

Don Piper reported standing at the gates of heaven and being over whelmed with dazzling colors. He saw streets of gold and gates of iridescent pearl. And every moment Don was in heaven he felt an intense love like he'd never experienced before.

Heaven will include streams of pure cool living water and trees bearing perfect fruit. Every where one looks there will be unimagined colors and beauty. Death and time will have passed away, but we will be active in praising and worshipping God as well as working in activities that bring us pure joy. Wow! I can't wait!

Paul kind of summarizes all of this in 1 Corinthians where he says in 1 Corinthians 2:9, "*However, as it is written: No eye has seen, nor ear has heard, no mind has conceived what God has prepared for those who love him.*"

Is there anyone reading this who would risk missing the above because of a lack of faith, laziness, self-centeredness, prohibited earthly pleasures, or any other hindrance? The Apostle Paul had it exactly right. He saw with clarity who Jesus was, and what lay ahead.

He put aside everything to attain the crown at the end of the race and I'm sure he ran right into the arms of God when he died and heard God say, "Well done good and faithful servant – nice race."

We too should have Paul's mindset. Nothing we experience here should keep us from running the race full out to the very end. As we've discussed earlier, running the race well actually will keep us healthier and provide longer life than if we slowed down and coasted to the finish line. So as Paul tells us in 1 Corinthians 9:24-27, *"...Run in such a way as to get the prize. Everyone who competes in the games goes into strict training ... we do it to get a crown that will last forever. Therefore I do not run like a man running aimlessly; I do not fight like a man beating the air. No, I beat my body and make it my slave so that after I have preached to others, I myself will not be disqualified for the prize."*

Paul is not the only one advising us on this. Listen to the following:

James 1:12, *"Blessed is the man who preservers under trial, because when he has stood the test, he will receive the crown of life that God has promised to those who love him."*

1 Peter 5:4, *"And when the Chief Shepherd appears, you will receive the crown of glory that will never pass away."*

Revelations 2:10, *"...Be faithful, even to the point of death, and I will give you the crown of life."*

Note this last scripture, which is God speaking through the Apostle John to the church at Smyrna, says be faithful "even to the point of death." There is no stopping here, no walking, no relaxing; it's serving to our last breath. That's what God wants.

Our time on earth is so short compared to eternity it would be a shame if we missed eternity because we blew it here. And the last third of our lives will be counted in the tally at the end of the race. The last third may determine whether the race is won or lost and, if we win, the treasures we store up in the last third will accrue to our heavenly account. Run well friend, run hard, and run to win!

I would now like to take a look at what churches and other Christian organizations might do to structure programs and activities to stimulate seniors to run their races not too but **"Thru The Tape."**

Chapter 11 - Senior Ministry
The Force to Guide Us

**Life is Like
Tennis – Serve
Well and You Win**

Can you envision the impact the rapidly growing population of Christian seniors could have on our country and world if they all attacked life as did Caleb (Joshua 14) discussed in chapter 2? If seniors followed the example of Caleb the Christian church could gain a new army of energetic workers to do good works and spread the gospel. The church could enlist an army of seniors who are "bearing fruit" and "staying fresh and green," and who could infuse the church with a new level of energy and excitement.

Before discussing what I believe the church must do, let's take a look at the demographics facing the church in the years ahead. As was mentioned earlier, the current attitude toward seniors was developed and conditioned by circumstances of the past. For example, in 1900 the life expectance at birth was 47 years. By the way it is still 47 years or less in many third world countries where AIDS and other health problems kill many adults and children early in life.

In the U.S.A. by the year 2000 our life expectancy had risen to 77. We added 30 years in one century. Some project a life expectancy of 125 by the year 2050. What we are certain of is that people are living longer than ever before. Better nutrition, better medical services, scientific advancements and other factors have added years to our lives.

While we have added years to our lives the retirement mentality we have hasn't changed since the Social Security (SS) system was put in place back in the 1930s. We assume people will work until 62-65 and then retire to a life of leisure before dying. The changing demographics, however, are putting SS in jeopardy. Instead of dying before retirement or soon after, which was the case when the system was put in place (life expectancy in 1930 was 57) people are now living another 15-20 years or more. This fact is taxing the SS financially, but it presents a tremendous opportunity for the church.

Here are some important statistics regarding our aging population taken from a recently released study by the Federal Interagency Forum on Aging-related Statistics.[13]

- In 2006, an estimated 37 million people in the U.S.A. were 65 and older roughly 12 % of the population. By 2030 projections are that there will be 71.5 million people 65 and over representing 20% of the population.

- In 2007, 76% of those 65 and over had a high school degree and 19% had at least a bachelor's degree.

---

[13] *Older Americans 2008: Key Indicators of Well-being*, Federal Interagency Forum on Aging-Related Statistics. (This is a group of 15 Federal agencies that use or produce data on older Americans. Their web site is at: www.agingstats.gov).

- In 2006, 9% of those 65 or over lived below the poverty line while those with high incomes were 29% of the group. (Up from 18% in a 1974 study).

- Older people, especially women, continue to work past 55 (more than in the past studies).

- The percent of older people who are obese is 31%, an increase from 22% in an earlier study completed in 1994.

- On an average day, most Americans age 65 and over spent at least half of their leisure time watching TV. Americans age 75 and older spent a higher proportion of their leisure time reading, relaxing and thinking than did those aged 55 to 64.

So what can we learn from these statistics? We see that the senior population is growing, is better educated, is more financially secure, but is out of shape and not using it's time wisely. So what can the church do? How does all this impact the church? I believe there is an army here for the church to enlist for the good of the seniors, for the good of the church, for the good of our communities, and for the good of God's kingdom. We can also assume that there are a large number of seniors, who either do not know the Lord and must come to know Him, and/or also there are many seniors who are living Christian lives but not at the level they should to achieve all the joy and happiness possible in their last years.

So how do we enlist this army? I believe the church is in the best position to both meet the needs of the seniors and to marshal this new army for the benefit of God's Kingdom. However, to do this there are several things the church needs to do to make it possible. Here's what I believe the church should do:

1. The church needs to change its attitudes about seniors. Seniors should be seen as productive mainstream church members who have a great deal to offer the church and community. The attitude that they can't be active or contribute must be changed. The church should view seniors as a valuable resource that can grow and increase, if seniors are challenged to stay active and productive.

2. The church should have an active educational program to educate and challenge seniors to grow, develop, and serve. Seniors need to know what the Bible says about aging and how to stay "fresh and green." They also need to have information on health, finances, death and dying, and other matters related to their age group to deal effectively with the issues they face. A progressive educational program of this type would also be offered to those approaching the retirement years so they can better prepare for them.

3. As part of the education program, seniors should be challenged to review their gifts, values, and experience and to consider how it can all be used in God's work in their senior years. There are programs available for helping seniors do this. Perhaps the best program in this area is called S.H.A.P.E. That means Spiritual gifts, Heart, Abilities, Personality, and Experience. The program has been developed by Rev. Erik

Rees, Pastor of Ministry at Saddleback Community Church in California. The program is outlined in his book entitled *Finding and Fulfilling Your Unique Purpose*. S.H.A.P.E. helps individuals inventory the blessings God has given them and how they might best fit into his kingdom's work. Such a program can also be custom designed for a church by a counselor or psychologist who may be a church member. In short, seniors need a well designed program to look inside in-depth to see what God has equipped them to best do in his kingdom's work. It is in finding this out that every senior will find the place where God wants them and where they can serve with ease and success. Remember Jesus has told us "My yoke is easy." It will only be easy if we find where he has equipped us to serve.

4. The church needs an energetic pastor or leader to serve as head of the program. Seniors have the capacity to run and pay for their own programs and activities but they need a leader in the church's leadership council to represent them, advocate for them, and to coordinate their activities.

5. In cases where churches are small in number, or have few seniors, churches should consider forming a senior group between churches, even if they must cross denominational lines to do it.

6. There needs to be a senior center in the church where seniors can go and meet together. This center needs to be open on a

regular scheduled basis and be a place a senior can go anytime to have a cup of coffee, meet a friend, use a computer, or play a table game. This center could be where the senior ministry pastor is officed and be a center of senior activities. Below you will find a list of the types of activities seniors might like to engage in and in the next chapter you will find more information on what a Christian senior center might look like in a church.

7. The church should be committed to having at least one Sunday worship service that is senior friendly. This means having music at a reasonable decibel level with some hymns and historic church music. Seniors should be made to feel they are a vital part of the congregation. If the church has a "blended" service combining newer praise music and hymns, the services must be balanced or seniors will feel like second class members.

Churches have an opportunity to help Christians not only prepare for their senior years but they should provide activities that facilitate and stimulate an active senior life. In Chapter 3 we mentioned the *Masterpiece Living Program* developed by the Mayo Clinic and the University of Michigan. They develop programs for seniors in four broad areas namely the mental, physical, social, and spiritual areas. I would add a fifth namely the volunteer area. In short, I believe churches should consciously develop a range of programs with a variety for seniors to choose from in each of the five areas. Later I will suggest a further refinement of this into a program called Caleb's Club to add some structure and fun to a comprehensive program.

It should be added here again that given the resources controlled by seniors (one study by AARP indicated that seniors control 70% of the discretionary income in the USA) they are entirely capable of paying for any facilities and programs they need. In fact, if seniors have their needs met, they will gladly and generously fund the vast majority of other church programs, including those of the children and youth.

Below are just some illustrations of the types of activities that might appeal to seniors along with the broad area into which the activity might fit.

Programs

The list is not exhaustive nor suggesting that they should all be included in such a program.

Senior Activities

	Activity	Value
1.	Book Club	Mental and Social Exercise
2.	Walking Club	Physical and Social Exercise
3.	Prayer Circle	Mental and Spiritual Exercise
4.	Aerobics Club	Physical and Social Exercise
5.	Knitting Club	Social and Volunteer Exercise
6.	Bible Study Group	Spiritual and Social Exercise

7.	Genealogy Group	Mental and Social Exercise
8.	Current Event Discussion Group	Mental and Social Exercise
9.	Travel and Mission Trip Club	Social and Volunteer Exercise
10.	Shut-in Visitation Group	Social and Volunteer Exercise
11.	Bowling Club	Physical and Social Exercise
12.	Golf Club	Physical and Social Exercise
13.	Stamp Collectors Club	Mental and Social Exercise
14.	Fix-it Club	Social and Volunteer Exercise
15.	Computer Club	Mental and Social Exercise
16.	Volleyball Club	Physical and Social Exercise
17.	Softball Club	Physical and Social Exercise
18.	Wellness Club	Physical and Social Exercise
19.	Volunteer's Club	Social and Volunteer Exercise
20.	Diner's Club	Social Exercise
21.	Bridge Club	Mental and Social Exercise
22.	Culinary Club	Social Exercise
23.	Investment Club	Mental and Social Exercise
24.	Garden Club	Physical and Social Exercise
25.	Fine Arts Club	Mental and Social Exercise
26.	Quilting Club	Social and Agility Exercise
27.	Cultural Study Club	Mental and Social Exercise
28.	Chess Club	Mental and Social Exercise
29.	Swim Club	Physical and Social Exercise
30.	Widows Support Group	Social and Volunteer Exercise
31.	Senior Chorus	Social and Volunteer Exercise
32.	Instrumental Group	Social and Volunteer Exercise
33.	Monopoly Group	Mental and Social Exercise

Caleb's Club

If a church wanted to go a step further than just having a senior ministry I would like to challenge them to develop a Caleb's Club or group with a special identification that would help the seniors to take a step of faith forward and serve God at a significant level in their senior years. Naming such a group after Caleb, that wonderful example of a vigorous dedicated servant of God, (see Joshua 14) would be a constant reminder of how seniors ought to deal with the last third of life. Note that the Caleb's Club proposed below is built on both the biblical principles and the scientific principles listed earlier in chapters 2 and 3. This club would have some similarities to the *Masterpiece Living Program* developed by the Mayo Clinic, the University of Michigan and others mentioned in chapter 3.

Such a club might have some special requirements for membership as illustrated below.

In order to be a member in good standing each year a senior in the Caleb's Club would sign a one year commitment to do the following:

1. Volunteer to participate regularly in at least one Christian ministry in the church or community.
2. Attend a weekly Bible study group.
3. Develop an individualized exercise program involving no less than exercise at least three times a week for 30 minutes each session.
4. Maintain a Body Mass Index of 30 or below.

5. Agree to have an individual daily devotion at least five days a week.

6. Attend at least one workshop or seminar a year covering a topic related to senior living.

7. Engage in at least one activity a day that would qualify as a mental exercise.

8. Commit to at least one activity weekly that involves a regular social component.

Seniors in such a program would develop individualized plans each year with the director of the program. This would allow for accommodating unique interests, abilities, and levels of aging. Programs for the Young Old (50-64), would differ from those of the Old (65-75) and from those of the Oldest (76+).

A Caleb's Club could do wonderful things together in terms of volunteering, meeting emergencies in the church and community and being an active force for good. If such a group was organized in a church I would hope they would be regularly recognized for their contributions and possibly even have a pin or other visible indication that they were proud members of Caleb's Club.

Can you imagine the energy and benefit that might accrue to the seniors, church, and community if all or a major share of the church's seniors belonged to a Caleb's Club? I think it would energize a church's seniors to do great things for God's kingdom.

The name isn't critical but I think calling it Caleb's Club would be a constant reminder of how one of God's favorite people lived his life and senior years. By following Caleb's example seniors can help insure, that as the Bible mentions, we will die at a "good old age."

Summary

It would be easy for a mega-church to develop a program such as described above; however, a comprehensive program could serve those even beyond the church membership. It has the potential for reaching into the senior population of a church's service area like nothing else could. It has the potential for reaching the un-churched for Christ and for marshalling volunteer resources to go out into the schools, hospitals, nursing homes, and charities in a church's community to minister in Christ's name. If a church wants to be a progressive church in the 21st century, which sets the example for others, rather than following, the church needs to get out front in planning a program something like that outlined above. To deny the demographics that are developing and to deny the needs of a growing senior population is to put our heads in the sand. Happily meeting the needs of seniors can create a wonderful synergy that will breathe new life and resources into the church and Christ's work everywhere.

An important part of a successful senior program should be a Christian senior center. Let's now take a look at what such a center might look like and how one might be developed in churches of various sizes.

Chapter 12 – The Christian Senior Center

Growing Old is Inevitable,
Living Old is a Choice
- Charles Stanley

In order to facilitate a fully developed senior ministry I believe a senior center of some type should be developed, and the most likely place to do that is in the church. It is important that seniors have a place to go regularly that is their "turf" and a place they can come to socialize, study, and serve. Most Christian seniors enjoy going to church and because most churches have spaces that are not highly used during the day, when seniors are most likely to use them, it is a natural place for them to focus their activity.

Seniors, as they grow older, may hesitate to leave their homes. There is a tendency for them to hibernate and become secluded. A vital senior center where they can count on meeting friends and having a good time is an important vehicle to get them out, active, and involved. The senior center doesn't have to be large and expensive but it does have to be well designed, comfortable, and planned for seniors.

Community Christian Senior Center

If one lives in a Christian community where most of the citizens are Christians it might be possible to develop a senior center for the community as a whole either in a mega-church or as a standalone facility. One such center now exists in Holland, Michigan and it is a wonderful success story. The Evergreen Commons is a senior center developed with the help of foundation funding and is built around a remodeled former Christian high school. The facilities and programs are comprehensive and are presently actually undergoing expansion. If you'd like to learn more about the Evergreen Commons you can go to the internet at www.evergreencommons.org. This web site also includes a layout of all of the facilities included in the complex which is located near the center of Holland.

Evergreen is open to all seniors in Western Michigan for a small annual fee and while it is open to all it has a strong Christian environment which includes a Christian chaplain. Evergreen Commons also has a program for senior adult daycare.

Many communities around the country have public senior centers. Some are successful and others are not well used. I believe a Christian senior center in a church has a better chance of serving the needs of seniors for several reasons. First, I believe Christian seniors like to go to their churches. It's a place where they feel comfortable. Second, Christian seniors ought to be motivated to meet together with other Christian seniors to study and serve their God. This is an aspect not often found in a public senior center. I also believe seniors will be attracted to a Christian senior center in a church where a wide variety of exciting and stimulating activities can be carried out to keep them "fresh and green." The Christian senior center can also be a place where the seniors invite non-Christian friends and it can be used as a base for evangelism and outreach.

The advantage of having a senior center in a church is that many of the facilities seniors might use are already there and many churches are not well used at the times seniors would normally use them, namely, during weekdays between 9:00 AM and 3:00 PM. Meeting rooms are usually available, and an auditorium for speakers and large group activities is there, as are kitchen facilities and restrooms. In short, churches are well suited to develop Christian senior centers.

Mega-churches have even more possibilities as many have gyms or multi-purpose facilities for physical activities, libraries, and even cafeterias or other eating facilities. A comprehensive senior ministry can easily be built around facilities that already exist.

Let me now list some of the functional areas that could be a part of a Christian senior center. Not all of them need to be in every center and a larger center in a mega-church will obviously have more than would a smaller church. After defining some of the functional areas I will present a couple of sample layouts of Christian senior centers one for a smaller church and one for a larger church setting. A senior center could include the following elements:

1. A reception area and an office for the senior ministry head and his/her support.

2. A coffee Kletz where seniors could meet their friends and socialize in an informal setting. This area might be in

conjunction with some lounge furniture where seniors could meet and discuss issues with their friends and where small groups might meet.

3. A computer area where seniors could learn to use computers and have access to the internet.

4. A game area where seniors could play table games or work on puzzles with their friends and get stimulating mental exercise.

5. An area with a large screen TV for viewing a variety of media materials including video exercise programs and games involving physical and mental exercises.

6. A meeting area for Bible study, workshops, and seminars. This area could be a regular classroom and hopefully have equipment for audio/visual presentations.

7. A library or reading area with books and materials of interest to seniors.

8. An arts and crafts room or area.

9. A music room for vocal and instrumental practice.

10. A gift shop or area for sale of items of interest to seniors.

11. A café or sandwich shop area for serving lunches.

12. A physical fitness area for individual exercising with proper equipment.

The planning and financing of a Christian senior center can and should be developed in conjunction with the seniors who will use it. The happy circumstance of working with seniors is they have the time, the skills, and the money to develop and fund their own programs.

They also know what needs they have and how they can best be met in a comprehensive senior ministry and center.

Seniors would be happy to help raise funds for such a center and, in fact, some of the fund raising projects could well help the seniors stay "fresh and green." Hymn sings, gospel concerts, yard sales, art sales, bake sales, and craft shows are just a few of the possible activities that could help raise money. If the seniors are allowed to brainstorm ways to raise the funds, I am sure they could come up with many ideas; in fact, the whole process could be a lot of fun for them.

There may be some communities where local philanthropists might contribute to a senior center and the possibility of foundation grants should be explored particularly if a senior daycare program is included.

Below you will find some renderings of possible senior centers in churches. They are presented to stimulate thinking and to show ideas of what is possible. The first rendering is of a Christian senior center in a small church that might have a large room that could be converted to a senior center during the week and yet be used at night or on Sundays for Sunday school class rooms or other activities.[14]

While the facilities below are shown in church buildings it is entirely possible to create the Christian senior center in a standalone

---

[14] Note – The renderings here have been developed by Mr. Ed Vermuslen A.I.A., NCARB, a Christian architect, and are used with his permission. Vermurlen Architecture is located at 5090 60th St. SE, Grand Rapids, MI 49512

building on the church grounds or as a wing or addition to the current church building.

So view the following material as information presented to help interested people develop ideas about what is possible and to be stimulated to become creative about developing their unique senior center.

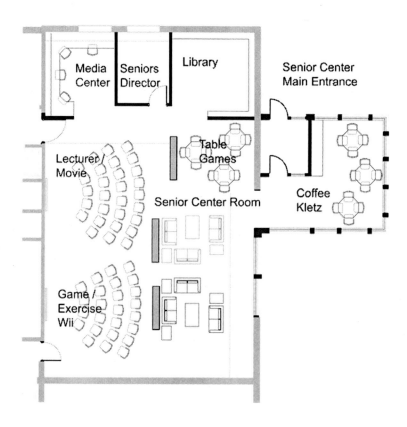

SENIOR CENTER
FIRST FLOOR PLAN PARTIAL
Small church example

In a smaller church the senior center would serve as a catalyst for senior activities and a place for seniors to gather. Some of the activities might be more easily held in homes or other church facilities. Bible studies, book reviews, discussions, and special speakers could be held here and it could be a regular meeting place where seniors would feel comfortable hanging out.

The high tech future holds the possibility of more opportunities for seniors to be entertained and stimulated mentally and physically at the same time.

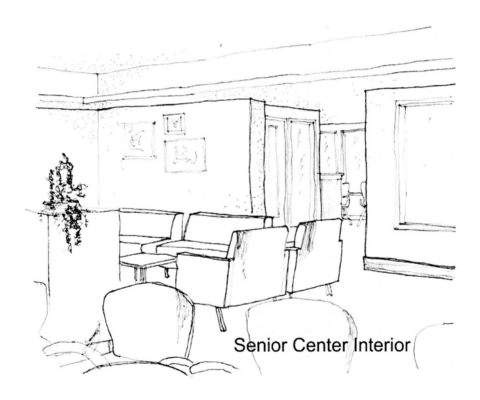

Senior Center Interior

This rendering shows a view from inside the senior center. The facility should be comfortably furnished and be a place that is attractive to further encourage seniors to go there and "hangout" with their friends. It should be a place where seniors would want to invite their non-Christian friends to come to have a good time as well as to socialize, learn, and grow.

The center can also be a place from which groups go out to serve others in the community and return to share their experiences.

A coffee kletz can be an important part of the center and the place where seniors can drop-in at any time to meet friends and socialize. The interior should have the "feel" of a comfortable living room environment. A nice addition to the room or kletz, if possible, would be a fireplace which would add warmth to the atmosphere particularly in the northern states in the winter.

In a large church or mega-church the opportunity to develop a comprehensive senior center and program are exceptional. A gym or multi-purpose room is nearly always available for recreational and exercise activities during the day. The auditorium or worship center is available for speakers and/or concerts and special events. Class rooms are available for Bible studies and club meetings even outside the senior center itself. If the group has a choir or instrumental groups there are rooms available for practice. Again many of the facilities needed by the senior program are already available at hours when they are currently not being used.

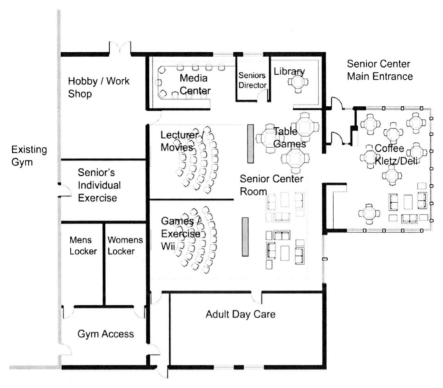

SENIOR CENTER
FIRST FLOOR PLAN PARTIAL
Large church example

Most of the facilities in the renderings above are self explanatory but one needs to be expanded upon because of the newness of it and the potential for the future. An area labeled in the renderings above is "Games/Exercise Wii" and has a great potential. Nintendo the electronic games maker has developed a series of games played on large screen TVs. It's called the Wii and uses wireless technology allowing for a wide range of activities. For example one can bowl, play baseball, and engage in many other games by standing

127

in front of the TV screen with a wireless gadget in ones hand and by emulating the movements made in playing that sport. This provides exercise and requires skill to do well.

A senior program with a Wii program could actually have a bowling league right in the senior center. Seniors could have teams, get exercise, and have fun all at the same time. The game keeps score and enough skill is needed for it to be interesting. Seniors could also play other games or use the area to exercise using a TV based exercise program designed for seniors. In short, for a relatively low cost the senior center could provide an exciting program that would attract seniors to the center for physical activity and social interaction.

As technology develops rapidly in the years to come it is fair to assume more things like Wii will develop that will provide a combination of activities to help seniors stay active mentally, physically, and socially. the senior center is a good place to provide such opportunities since many would be unable financially to afford them in their homes.

Senior Adult Daycare

One of the growing areas of need in the country due to the growing number of older senior citizens is for elder daycare. As seniors live longer, and as many are being cared for by their children many of whom are working, there is a need for a service where seniors who need special care might be taken during the day. Eldercare centers are developing all across America even as childcare centers developed several decades ago.

Many of these centers are being developed in or in conjunction with churches. If a church develops a Christian senior center it might be wise to also consider developing an adult daycare center as well. One should be warned, however, that developing such a center carries with it the responsibility for meeting a host of state and federal requirements and the facilities must meet special standards. There are grants available for developing such centers and there are foundations with a heart for such programs. As seniors increase in number and live much longer, these types of facilities will be needed more. An eldercare facility can, as with children's daycare programs, develop a profit over time and be a self supporting function. It is a natural adjunct to a senior center and has developed as such at the Evergreen Commons mentioned above.

Summary

And so ends the discussion of how I believe God wants us to finish the race of life by "Running Thru the Tape." The last part of life can be the best and it can end happily and productively for all who are "called according to God's purposes." I pray the scriptures cited, the examples given, and the reasoning outlined will convince every senior reading this book that the best can still be ahead, because that has been the experience of my wife and me.

You will find some additional material in the appendices that follow which I hope will be of interest and value. There are over 200 web sites listed that have value for seniors, an appendix on senior humor, and some forms that may be helpful in planning.

If you would like to learn more about me and/or to communicate with me you can do so by going to my web site at: www.sentencesermons.com.

Appendix A - Web Sites For Seniors

The Internet contains a wealth of information for seniors. There are millions of web sites that provide information that can be helpful as well as entertaining and the technology is getting better all the time. Someone recently estimated that 100,000 new web sites are added to the Internet every week. Once one has a computer and an Internet connection you can go to the various web sites free of charge and have the world of information and knowledge at your finger tips. Even if one doesn't have a computer you can often use one for free that is connected to the Internet at your local library though they may limit the time used per visit.

Arts and Entertainment	
Art Museum and Gallery Guide	
Movies (Times and locations of local movies)	www.moviefone.com
Playbill Online (Lists what is playing on Broadway and elsewhere.)	www.playbill.com
Associations and Senior Sites	
Administration on Aging (federal agency responsible for administration of Older Americans Act)	www.aoa.dhhs.gov
American Association of Retire Persons (AARP)	www.aarp.org
National Council on Aging	www.ncoa.org
Senior Search (Information linked to Canada and Australia)	www.seniorsearch.com

Seniors-Site (A wealth of information in links to other sites)	www.artinfo.com/galleryguide
Significant Living (An organization for Christian seniors)	www.significantliving.org
Beds and Breakfasts	
The Inn-Guide (Includes 50 states and beyond)	www.inn-guide.com
Book Buying Online	
Amazon	www.amazon.com
Barnes and Noble	www.barnesandnoble.com
Christian Books	www.christianbook.com www.kregel.com www.readingup.com
Cartoons	
Free cartoons for fun and laughter	www.glasbergen.com
Charities and Giving	
Better Business Bureau (Rates charities against acceptable standards)	www.bbb.org
Charity Watch (Rates charities)	www.charitywatch.org
Evangelical Council for Financial Accountability	www.ecfa.org
National Charities Information (Online guide to 400 charities)	www.give.org
Christian Sites	
American Family Association	www.afa.net
Christian News	www.cnsnews.com
Christianity Today (with links to other sites)	www.christianity.net
Religious Information	www.crosswalk.com

Dating Services	
Dating Services for Christians	www.eharmony.com www.seniorfriendfinder.com
Dictionary	
Free Dictionary	www.onelook.com
Directories	
Telephone listings for more than 100 million individuals and businesses in the United States	www.switchboard.com
Zip Code directory and address information	www.usps.gov/ncsc
Education	
Elderhostel (Travel and learn with seniors)	www.elderhostel.org
New Promises (Take college courses online)	www.mindedge.com
Senior Net (Relates information technology to seniors; learn to use a computer)	www.seniornet.org
Elder Care	
Sites with information on elder care programs	www.elderweb.com www.elderlink.com www.eldercare.gov
Encyclopedias	
Online encyclopedias	www.britannica.com www.letsfindout.com www.wikipedia.org
Family Research (Genealogical Services)	
RootsWeb	www.rootsweb.ancestry.com
The USGenWeb Project	www.usgenweb.com

Financial Planners	
Crown Financial Ministries	www.crown.org
Dave Ramsey	www.daveramsey.com
Kingdom Advisors	www.kingdomadvisors.org
Financial Planning Association	www.fpanet.org
Flowers and Gardening	
Buy flowers online	www.ftd.com
Gardening	www.gardenmart.com
Plant Encyclopedia	www.gardening.com
Franchises	
American Franchise Association	www.franchise.org
Federal Trade Commission	www.ftc.gov
Government Services	
Federal Consumer Information Center	www.pueblo.gas.gov
Library of Congress (Indexed information on a wide variety of subjects	www.loc.gov
Social Security	www.ssa.gov
U.S. Treasury (Internal Revenue Service and other Treasury information and forms)	www.ustreas.gov www.irs.gov
Greeting Cards	
Blue Mountain Greeting Cards (Email free cards to friends)	www.bluemountain.com
Health Related Sites	
Health information and links	www.allhealth.com

Appendix A - Web Sites For Seniors

American Heart Association	www.americanheart.org
American Medical Association	www.ama-assn.org
Center for Disease Control	www.cdc.gov
The Fellowship of Merry Christians	www.joyfulnoiseletter.com
World Health Online	www.healthy.net
Mayo Clinic Health Information	www.mayoclinic.com
Medicare	www.medicare.gov
National Institutes of Health	www.nih.gov
Pain Control	www.pain.com
Women's Health	www.womenshealth.gov
WebMD	www.webmd.com
Insurance Information	
Insurance quotes (From competing companies)	www.quickquote.com www.insure.com
Investors Information	
Investors clubs and information	www.iclub.com
National Association of Investors	www.better-investor.org
The National Center for Home Equity Conversion (Information on reverse mortgages)	www.reverse.org
Best bulletin boards for stocks	www.investorvillage.com
Security and Exchange Commission (Company filings of financial reports)	www.sec.gov
The Universal Currency Converter	www.xe.net/ucc
Yahoo Finance (Information plus stock tracking – click Finance	www.yahoo.com

Jobs	
Find Christian jobs	www.christianjobs.com www.churchstaffing.com www.encorecareers.com
Legal Assistance	
National Senior Citizen Law Center	www.nsclc.org
Newspapers and Columnists	
Drudge Report (Latest news and links to major columnists)	www.drudgereport.com
Jerusalem Post	www.jpost.com
The New York Times	www.nytimes.com
USA Today	www.usatoday.com
The Washington Post	www.washingtonpost.com
Real Estate	
Homes for sale by owners	www.owners.com
Home Hunter (With links to ads in 31 daily newspapers)	www.homehunter.com
Realtor.com (Listings of over one million homes with mapping capability)	www.realtor.com
Search Engines on the Internet	
DogPile	www.dogpile.com
Google	www.google.com
HotBot	www.hotbot.com
Go	www.go.com
WebCrawler	www.webcrawler.com
Yahoo	www.yahoo.com

Appendix A - Web Sites For Seniors

Senior Living	
American Association of Homes and Services for the Aging	www.aahsa.com
American Health Care Association	www.ahcancal.org
Assisted Living Federation of America	www.alfa.org
National Association for Home Care and Hospice	www.nahc.org
Sports Information	
CBS Sports	www.sportsline.com
ESPN Sports Center	www.espn.go.com
Sports Competitions for Seniors	
National Senior Games Association	www.nsga.com
Over 50 Baseball Leagues	www.over50baseball.com
Rowing	www.usrowing.org
Swimming	www.usms.org
Track and Field	www.usatf.org
Travel	
Cheap Airline Tickets	www.cheaptickets.com
Elderhostel (Inexpensive travel and educational experiences with seniors)	www.elderhostel.org
Free maps and directions	www.mapsonus.com www.mapquest.com
Reasonable Travel Service	www.expedia.com
Bid on airline tickets	www.priceline.com
State Department travel warnings	www.travel.state.gov

Volunteer Opportunities for Seniors	
Christian Volunteers	www.christianvolunteering.org
Habitat for Humanity	www.habitat.org
Missionary Assistance Program	www.mmap.org
Prison Fellowship Ministry	www.pmf.org
Roving Volunteers	www.rvics.com
Senior Corps	www.seniorcorps.org
Service Corps of Retired Executives (SCORE)	www.score.org
Sower Ministry	www.sowerministry.org

Appendix B - Senior Humor

As mentioned earlier, humor and laughter is health producing. Humor has the potential for healing, for extending life, and for bringing a joy to life that few if any other forces can bring. Laughter can color life and make it more enjoyable. As someone once said, "We don't stop laughing because we grow old; we grow old because we stop laughing."

It is particularly healthy if people can learn to laugh at themselves. We just seem to get along better if we don't take ourselves too seriously. It is important for seniors to be able to laugh at themselves as well. Actually we can be very humorous at times. Below you will find some stories, jokes, and cartoons many aimed at seniors. Some of the stories you will have heard and others may be new. A good story like a good song deserves to be repeated. So read on, laugh some and I guarantee you will feel better.

Interspersed with some of the jokes are some cartoons from one of my favorite cartoonists Randy Glasbergen. His cartoons can be found on the internet at: www.glasbergen.com.

Senior Prayer – "So far today, God, I've done all right. I haven't gossiped, haven't lost my temper, haven't been selfish, nasty, grumpy, or over indulgent. I'm really glad about that. But in a few moments I'm going to get out of bed, and from then on I'm going to need all the help I can get. Please help me in Jesus name. Amen"

The Believer – A senior and a young man were shipwrecked on a Pacific Island. The young man was terribly upset and began screaming, "We're going to die, no one will ever find us." The senior gentleman sat calmly by under a palm tree and said nothing. The young man said to him, "Aren't you worried? We're going to die!" The senior said, "I'm not worried at all you see I am a Christian, I tithe, and I make over $100,000 a week. If we just sit by calmly, I'm sure my pastor will find us shortly."

Elephant Hunting – Why don't seniors go elephant hunting? The answer – Because they can't lift the decoys anymore.

The Cure – A lady was talking to a friend and said, "I've cured my husband from biting his nails." "How'd you do that?" her friend asked. "I hid his false teeth," she replied.

The Senior Golfer – A senior parishioner went golfing frequently with his pastor. The pastor never could beat the elderly gentleman no matter how hard he tried. One day the parishioner saw how depressed the pastor was that he couldn't beat him so to console him he said, "Don't worry pastor one of these days you will bury me." The pastor replied, "I know I will, but even then it will be your hole."

Speechless – Red Skelton, the comedian, was asked if there was ever a time when he was speechless. He said it had happened only once. He said he had a dream that he was brought before God. Just as he was introduced, God sneezed. Skelton said that for the first time in his life he didn't know what to say.

One's Age – A little boy asked his grandfather how old he was and the grandfather replied he wasn't quite sure. The little boy then replied that he should look in his underware because in his it said he was 4-6.

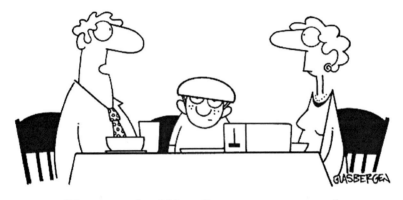

**"I'm not saying kids today are over-protected,
but *I* never had to wear a helmet to make toast!"**

The Lost Baby – A sixty five year old woman had a baby and some of her friends came over to see it. When the woman did not produce the baby, one of her friends asked if they could see it. The elderly woman said they could see the baby when the baby started to cry because she forgot where she left it.

Splitting the Meal – An elderly couple went to a Mc Donald's and got one meal which they then carefully split in two. A friend sitting nearby watched as the man began to eat his half of the meal but the wife didn't eat a bite. Finally the friend came over and asked the woman how come she wasn't eating her half of the meal. She replied that she would begin eating as soon as her husband was through using the teeth.

The Memory – A senior said to his elderly friend, "Did you know that our memories are the second thing to go?" "Is that right?" said the friend, "What's the first?" "I forgot," he replied.

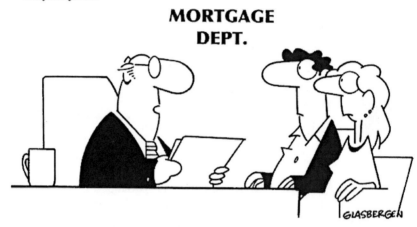

MORTGAGE DEPT.

"Your children are quite young and likely to wet the bed. Technically, that puts you in a flood zone so your interest rate would be higher."

The Math Test – A doctor had three Alzheimer's patients down at the retirement home. One Monday he visited them, got them together in a room, and decided to give them a math test to see how they were doing. First, he asked George how much 3x3 was. George thought for a moment and said 252. Next, the doctor asked John how much 3x3 was and he said Tuesday. Well the doctor was disappointed in the results but he continued by asking Sam how much 3x3 was. Sam said, nine. The doctor was thrilled that he had gotten it right and asked Sam how he had gotten his answer. Sam replied it was easy he just subtracted Tuesday from 252.

Lot's Wife – A grandfather was reading the Bible story of Lot to his grandson. He read that the man named Lot was warned to take his wife and flee out of the city, but she looked back and became a pillar of salt. "What happened to the flea?" asked his grandson.

The Ex-Marine – There was a professor at a large university who was an atheist and liked to show off to his class. One day he said to the class, "Today I'm going to prove to you there is no God. He walked out from behind his desk and said, "God, if you exist strike me down." When nothing happened he said, "See, there's no God," and again he repeated, "God if you exist strike me down." At this time an elderly gentleman and a former Marine came forward and hit the professor on the chin knocking him to the floor. The professor was stunned and he said, "Why did you do that?" The ex-Marine said, "God was busy so he sent me."

The Hereafter – A minister approached one of his senior parishioners and told him that he should be thinking about the hereafter. The man responded by saying that he was constantly thinking about the hereafter when he was in the kitchen, the garage, the bedroom, and the basement. He said "I'm always asking myself, now, what am I here after?"

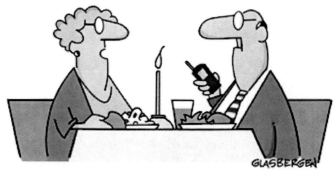

"You seem like a nice gentleman, but I'm not sure
I could ever get serious about a man who has
a laxative jingle for his ring tone."

Signs of Aging – You can get an indication you're getting old
if:

- You sit in a rocking chair and can't get it going.
- You burn the midnight oil starting at 8:00 P.M.
- You look forward to a dull evening.
- Your knees buckle and your belt won't.
- Your little black book contains only names ending in M.D.
- Your back goes out more than you do.
- You decide to procrastinate and never get around to it.
- You walk with your head held high trying to get used to your bifocals.
- You sink your teeth into a steak and they stay there.

- More hair is growing in your nose and ears than on your head.

- It takes longer to rest than to get tired.

- Caution is the only thing you care to exercise.

- Work is less fun and fun is more work.

- You mind makes contracts your body can't keep.

- You call the Incontinence Hotline and they tell you to please hold.

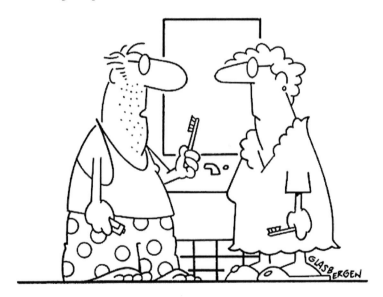

© Randy Glasbergen.
www.glasbergen.com

"Look at the bright side. It's nice to know that our sex life doesn't contribute to global warming."

The Wrong Way – A senior lady was pulled over by a policeman for going the wrong way on a busy one-way street. The policeman said, "Lady don't you know you're going the wrong way?" She replied, "Well, I guess it doesn't matter it looks like everyone else is coming back anyway."

The Energy Efficient Vehicle – A man pulled up behind an elderly Amish couple in their horse drawn carriage. On the rear he saw a sign that read: Energy Efficient Vehicle – Runs on Oats and Grass – Don't Step on the Exhaust.

The Four Husbands – An elderly lady was being interviewed by a radio announcer and he asked her if she was married. She said she was and had had four husbands. When asked what her husbands' occupations were she said, "The first was a banker, the second was a ringmaster in the circus, the third was a preacher, and her current one was a mortician." The announcer then said, "That's a wide variety of occupations your husband's had." She responded, "There was one for the money, two for the show, three to get ready, and four to go."

The Crossword Puzzle – An elder lady was doing a crossword puzzle on an airplane and she had a problem with a word. She leaned over to a man sitting next to her and asked if he would help her with a word and he said he'd be glad to. She said the word was four letters and ended in "i-t." The definition says it's found on the bottom of a bird cage and the mayor of Detroit is full of it. The man thought for a moment and said the word was "grit." "Oh, yes," said the women, "so it is! Then she said, "By the way, do you have an eraser?"

The New Bride – An elderly widower brought home a new bride. His son took one look at her and pulled his father aside and whispered to him, "Dad, I've never seen such a homely woman, she has hair on her chin; her eyes are watching each other; and her teeth are crooked." "You don't have to whisper," said the father, "She's deaf too, but she can drive at night."

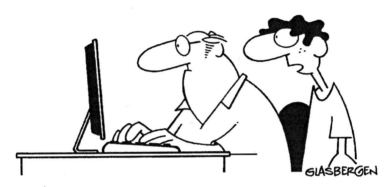

"There's nothing wrong with your blog, Dad.
I just don't think anyone wants to read
your ideas for styling ear hair."

The Intelligent Dog – A young man went to a movie and sat behind an elderly gentleman sitting next to a dog who was watching the movie. The dog was paying attention and waging his tail at appropriate times. The young man leaned over to the elderly gentleman and said he was amazed that the dog was so interested in the movie. The gentleman then said, "I'm surprised too, since he didn't like the book."

The Chess Match – A deliveryman entered a retirement home and saw a resident playing chess with a dog. He watched and saw the dog move the pieces, and bark when he achieved checkmate. Finally the deliveryman said to the elderly gentleman, "That's a brilliant dog,

I've never seen a dog play chess before." The man replied, "He's not so smart I beat him three out of four matches."

The Retort – An elderly man was pestering one of the handsome ladies at the retirement home. One day he was bothering her and leaned over to her saying, "Please say the three little words that will make me walk on air." She looked at him and said, "Go hang yourself."

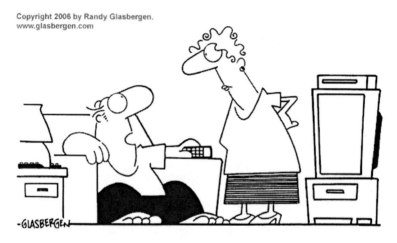

Copyright 2006 by Randy Glasbergen.
www.glasbergen.com

"I do so help around the house! I keep dust off the recliner and make sure all of the remotes are working properly!"

The Marriage – Grandpa Jones, who was 85, came home and announced he was going to marry a beautiful young lady who was 21 years old. His daughter said that she was deeply concerned because at his age that kind of a marriage could be dangerous, even fatal. Grandpa Jones responded by saying he realized it was dangerous, but if she died, she died.

The Hair Dye – An elderly woman went into a beauty salon and told the operator that she wanted her hair dyed back to its original color. "What color was that," she was asked. "I don't remember," she replied.

The Chewing Gum – An elderly lady was taking her first airplane ride and as the plane descended her ears began to hurt due to the change in air pressure. She called a cabin attendant over and said her ears were hurting and asked if there was anything she could do. The attendant said, "Yes, just chew this piece of gum and everything should be O.K." As they were leaving the plane the attendant asked the elderly lady if her ears were alright. The lady said, "My ears are fine, now how do I get the gum out of them?"

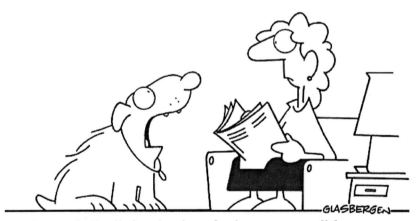

"First my ball rolled under the sofa, then my water dish was too warm, then the squeaker broke on my rubber pork chop. I've had a horrible day and I'm totally stressed out!!!"

The Sunday Paper - An irate senior citizen called her local newspaper to complain bitterly about the fact that she hadn't received her Sunday newspaper. "Where's my Sunday paper?" she said, "It's usually here by now." The lady at the paper said, "Madam this is Saturday, we don't deliver the paper until tomorrow which is Sunday. "Oh crap," the lady was heard to mutter, "That's why there wasn't anyone in church today."

The Big Mouth – An elderly couple were pulled over by a policeman. He walked to the car window and said to the man who was driving, "I clocked you going 70 MPH in a 50 MPH zone." The man's wife sitting next to him said, "Oh, no, officer, he was doing 80 MPH. Then the officer said, "I'm also going to have to ticket you for not wearing your seat belt." The man said, "Officer, I had it on and just took it off as you came to the window." The man's wife said, "That's not true, officer, he never wears his seat belt." Then the policeman said, "I'm also going to have to ticket you for your broken tail light." The man said, "But, officer, it was just broken this morning and I'm on my way to the dealer to get it fixed." His wife then said, "That's not true, officer, the tail light has been broken for six months." At that, the man lost it and yelled at his wife, "Can't you keep your big mouth shut." The officer then said to the woman, "Does he always yell at you like that?" "No," she replied, "He only yells at me like that when he's drunk."

The Bad Speller – An elderly gentleman had struggled with spelling all of his life. He just could not spell very well. One day his wife fell down and injured herself. The man quickly called 911 and said he needed an ambulance to take his wife to the hospital. "Where do you live?" asked the operator. "We live on Eucalyptus Street," replied the elder gentleman. "Would you please spell that for me?" asked the operator. There was a long pause on the phone. Finally the man responded by saying, "Would it be all right if I dragged my wife over to Oak St.?"

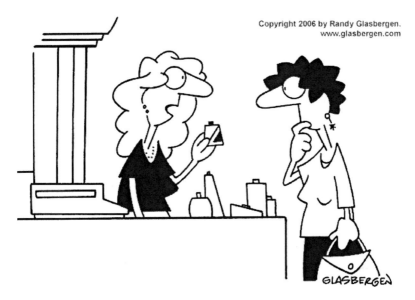

GLASBERGEN

"Men love this scent! It smells like electronics sprayed with car exhaust then dipped in BBQ sauce!"

The Naughty Parrot – An elderly gentleman bought a parrot for a pet. When he got it home the parrot started insulting the gentleman and was using foul language. The man said if he didn't stop he'd punish him. The parrot kept on so the elderly gentleman put the parrot in the refrigerator. The parrot continued swearing but then suddenly stopped. The man took him out and the parrot apologized profusely for his bad behavior. The man accepted the apology. The parrot then said, "If you don't mind my asking, what did that chicken in there do?"

The Wise Farmer – A farmer had a pond near his farm house but he was too busy to go there very often. One day he heard a lot of noise at the pond and when he went to see what it was he found several young girls skinny dipping. When they saw him they went to the deep end and said they would not come out until he left. The farmer said he wouldn't bother them and that he had only come down to the pond to feed the alligator. Moral – Old age and trickery will overcome youth and skill every time.

The Hippy – An elderly gentleman was sitting in a mall having coffee when a young hippy came and sat near him. The young man had his hair spiked and dyed different colors. Every time the young man looked at the gentleman he was staring at him. Finally the young man said sarcastically, "What's the matter old man, haven't you ever done anything crazy in your life?" The gentleman replied, "Yes I have. Once when I was young I got very drunk and became intimate with a peacock. I was just wondering if you might be my son."

The Elderly Sisters – Three elderly sisters 92, 94, and 96 lived together. One day the 96 year old had one foot in the bath tub and one out and asked her 94 year old sister if she would come and tell her if she was getting in or out of the tub because she had forgotten. The 94 year old got part way up the stairs and forgot whether she was going up or down so she called to her younger sister to come and tell her if she was going up or down. The younger sister who was sitting at the kitchen table said to herself thank goodness I'm not that forgetful and to reinforce it she knocked on wood. She then responded to her sister that she would be there in a minute as soon as she found out who was knocking at the door.

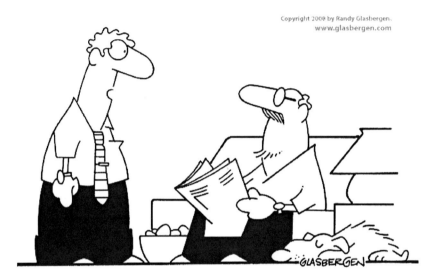

"Sorry, I've never been very good at remembering names, Mom."

Quips about Old Age

You know you're old when the candles on your birthday cake resemble a raging forest fire.

I don't feel 80; in fact, I don't feel anything until noon. Then it's time for my nap. – **Bob Hope**

She was so old that when she went to school they didn't have history. – **Rodney Dangerfield**

Anyone can get old. All you have to do is live long enough. – **Groucho Marx**

I've found the secret of youth. I lie about my age. – **Bob Hope**

When I get up in the morning the first thing I do is read the obituaries. If my name isn't there, I shave. – **George Burns**

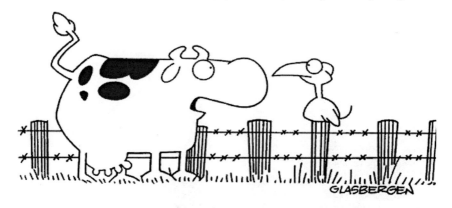

Copyright 1996 Randy Glasbergen.   www.glasbergen.com

**"It's true, I did jump over the moon.
I had waaaaay too much coffee that day!"**

Age is strictly a case of mind over matter. If you don't mind it doesn't matter. – **Jack Benny**

My doctor told me I look like a million dollars – green and wrinkled. – **Red Skelton**

One way to improve your memory is to lend people money

Don't worry about senility, my grandfather used to tell me. When it hits you, you'll never know it. – **Bill Cosby**

I'm at an age where my back goes out more than I do – **Phyllis Diller**

Appendix C - Advanced Directives

An advanced directive, sometimes called a living will, is a legal instrument which contains a person's wishes regarding a series of end-of-life issues including medical care.

The advanced directive is not to be confused with a person's will or trust arrangements which cover the distribution of one's estate. The advanced directive is in addition to the will and should be executed as a separate legal document to cover end-of-life issues not covered by the traditional will or trust arrangement.

On the following pages we have provided a sample of an advanced directive so you may see the kinds of issues that are covered. This document may be used by the reader; however, you should be aware that each state has requirements regarding the content and form of an advanced directive. These requirements should be consulted before executing such an instrument.

There is an organization called Aging with Dignity which has done some marvelous work in the area of advanced directives. Supported by the Robert Woods Foundation this organization has developed an advanced directive entitled Five Wishes. Five Wishes has been legally accepted in 40 states as a legal document. It has been carefully crafted through research with seniors and covers all of the major issues.

One can access the information regarding Five Wishes, including which states accept it as a legal instrument, by calling 888-594-7437 or by going to their web site at: www.agingwithdignity.org. They have a 25 minute video which explains the process and the document they have developed. There is a small charge for the materials they provide. Their mailing address is:

Aging with Dignity
P.O. Box 1661
Tallahassee, Florida 32302-1661

Advanced Directive[15]

My Durable Power of Attorney for Health Care, Living will, and Other Wishes.

I, _____, write this document as a directive regarding my medical care. (Put your initials below by the choices you want.)

Part 1. My durable Power of Attorney for Health Care.

I appoint the following person to make decisions about my medical care if there ever comes a time when I cannot make these decisions myself.

Name_____

Address_____

Home phone_____

Work phone_____

If the person above cannot or will not make decisions for me I appoint this person.

Name_____

Address_____

Home phone_____

_____

[15] Note: Because states differ in their language requirements, please consult an attorney before using this document.

Work phone_____

_____ I have not appointed anyone to make health care decisions for me in any other document.

_____ I want the person I have appointed, my doctors, my family, and others to be guided by decisions I have made in the following pages.

Part 2. My Living Will

These are my wishes for my future medical care if there ever comes a time when I cannot make these decisions for myself.

A. These are my wishes if I have a terminal condition.

Life-sustaining Treatments

_____ I do not want life-sustaining treatments (Including CPR). If life-sustaining treatments are administered, I want them stopped.

_____ I want life-sustaining treatments that my doctors think are best for me.

_____ Other wishes:_____

Artificial Nutrition and Hydration

_____ I do not want artificial nutrition and hydration started if it would be the main treatment keeping me alive. If artificial nutrition and hydration are started, I want them stopped.

_____ I do want artificial nutrition and hydration, even if it is the main treatment keeping me alive.

_____ Other wishes:_____

Comfort Care

_____ I want to be kept as comfortable and free of pain as possible, even if such care prolongs my dying or shortens my life.

_____ Other wishes: _____

B. These are my wishes if I am ever in a persistent vegetative state.

Life-sustaining Treatments

_____ I do not want life-sustaining treatments (including CPR). If life-sustaining treatments are administered, I want them stopped.

_____ I want life-sustaining treatments that my doctors think are best for me.

_____ Other wishes:_____

Artificial Nutrition and Hydration

_____ I do not want artificial nutrition and hydration started if it would be the main treatment keeping me alive. If artificial nutrition and hydration have been started, I want them stopped.

_____ I do want artificial nutrition and hydration, even if it is the main treatment keeping me alive.

_____ Other wishes:_____

Comfort Care

_____ I want to be kept as comfortable and free of pain as possible, even if such care prolongs my dying or shortens it.

C. Other Directions

(You have the right to be involved in all decisions about your medical care, even those not dealing with terminal conditions or a persistent vegetative state. If you have wishes not covered in other parts of this document, please indicate them here.)

Part 3. Other Wishes

1. Organ Donation

_____ I do not wish to donate my organs or tissue.

_____ I want to donate all of my organs and tissue.

_____ I want to donate only these organs and tissues: _____

_____

Other wishes: _____

2. Autopsy

_____ I do not want an autopsy.

_____ I agree to an autopsy if my doctors request it.

_____ Other wishes: _____

(If you wish to say more about any of the above choices, or if you have any other statements to make about your medical care, you may do so on a separate sheet of paper. If you should choose to add a statement, put here the number of pages you are adding. _____)

Part 4. Signatures

(In most states you and two witnesses must sign and date the advanced directive for it to be legal. There will be a paragraph above your signature that attests you understand the document. There will be a paragraph stating that your witnesses attest you are signing of your own free will. You will want to choose witnesses who are not related to you by blood, adoption, or marriage. Again consult an attorney for the requirements and language necessary in your state.)

Appendix D - A Dying Person's Bill of Rights[16]

1. I have the right to be treated as a living human being until I die.
2. I have the right to maintain a sense of hopefulness, however changing its focus may be.
3. I have the right to be cared for by those who can maintain a sense of hopefulness, however changing this may be.
4. I have the right to express my feelings and emotions about my approaching death in my own way.
5. I have the right to participate in decisions concerning my care.
6. I have the right to expect continuing medical and nursing attention, even though "cure" goals must be changed to "comfort" goals.
7. I have the right not to die alone.
8. I have the right to be free from pain.
9. I have the right to have my questions answered honestly.
10. I have the right not to be deceived.
11. I have the right to have help from and for my family in accepting my death.
12. I have the right to die in peace and with dignity.
13. I have the right to retain my individuality and not be judged for my decisions, which may be contrary to the beliefs of others.
14. I have the right to discuss my religious and/or spiritual experiences, whatever they may mean to others.

---

[16] Created at a hospice workshop on the terminally ill patient held in Lansing, MI.

15. I have the right to expect that the sanctity of the human body will be respected after death.

16. I have the right to be cared for by caring, sensitive, knowledgeable people who will attempt to understand my needs and will be able to gain some satisfaction in helping me face my death.

Appendix E - Financial Forms

1.   Family Net Worth Calculator

2.   Budget Form

3.   Family Cash Flow Projections – Monthly and Annual

Family Net Worth Calculator			
Assets	Current Value	**Liabilities**	Current Value
Cash		**Mortgages**	
Checking Account		Residence	
Savings Account/CDs		2nd Mortgage	
Money Mkt. Funds		Vacation Home	
		Invest. Property	
Total		Total	
Securities		**Other Debt**	
Stocks		Auto/boat Loans	
Bonds		Bank Loans	
Mutual Funds		Other Loans	
Total		Total	
Real Estate		**Consumer Debt**	
Residence		Credit Cards	
Vacation Home		Charge Accounts	
Investment Property		Other	
Total		Total	
Other Assets		**Taxes**	
Business Interests		Federal	
Debts Receivable		State/Local	
Vested Pension			
Collectibles			

Appendix E - Financial Forms

Life Ins. Cash Value			
Annuities Sur. Value			
IRAs, 401ks Value			
Others (List)			
Total		Total	
Personal		**Obligations**	
Automobiles		Other	
Home Furn./Jewelry		Miscellaneous	
Boat/Trailer			
Other:			
Other:			
Total		Total	
Total Assets		**Total Liabilities**	
Net Worth (Assets – Liabilities)			

Annual Family Budget

Most families on fixed incomes can benefit from developing a family budget in order to plan and control expenditures. Below you will find a budget form that also includes percentages expended by the average retired Christian family. While every family is unique these percentages will allow for comparison with others to see how your family matches up with other retired families. Such a comparison may allow for identification of areas where savings may be made. The percentages are approximations based on a national study of expenditures by retired families and have been adjusted for a Christian's tithe.

Expenditures[17]	Monthly	Annual	% of Budget
Food (12%)			
Housing (25%)			
Clothing (4%)			
Entertainment (4%)			
Healthcare (14%)			
Insurance (5%)			
Taxes (5%)			
Transportation (14%)			
Charity (10%)			
Utilities (5%)			
Other (2%)			
Total (100%)			

---

[17] Percentages represent those of an average retired Christian family that tithes. These figures have been modified slightly for a Christian family from figures developed in a national study of retired families.

Appendix E - Financial Forms

Cash Flow Projection

I. Income	Monthly	Annual
A. Wages/Salary (Gross)		
B. Interest/Dividents		
C. Other		
D. Other		
Total		
II. Expenses		
A. Mortgage		
B. Insurance (Home)		
C. House (Miscellaneous)		
D. Food		
E. Utilities (Gas, electricity, water)		
F. Telephone		
G. Cable TV		
H. Auto Insurance		
I. Gas and Oil		
J. Auto Repairs		
K. Clothing		
L. Giving (Church, charity)		
M. Entertainment		
N. Eating out		
O. Newspaper, Magazines		
P. Barber, hairdresser		
Q. Medical (Payments, insurance)		
R. Dental (Payments, insurance)		
S. Install. Pay. (Credit cards, debts)		
T. Taxes (Payroll, FICA)		
U. Vacation		
V. Other		
Total		
III. Cash Flow		
A. Income (Total from I. above)		
B. Expenses (Total from II above)		
Cash Flow (A minus B)		

Other Titles From
Dr. L. James Harvey

701 Sentence Sermons
(Grand Rapids, Michigan: Kregel Publications, 2000)

701 More Sentence Sermons
(Grand Rapids, Michigan: Kregel Publications, 2002)

701 Sentence Sermons - Volume 3
(Grand Rapids, Michigan: Kregel Publications, 2005)

701 Sentence Sermons - Volume 4
(Grand Rapids, Michigan: Kregel Publications, 2007)

Every Day Is Saturday
(St. Louis, Missouri: Concordia Publishing House, 2000)

The Resurrection - Ruse or Reality?
(Baltimore, Maryland: Publish America, 2001)

The Resurrection on Trial
(A play based on the book above - Self published by Dr. Harvey and available for purchase from him at www.sentencesermons.com)

Letters from Perverse University
(Lincoln, Nebraska: Author's Choice Press, 2001)

Seven For Heaven
(Lima, Ohio: CSS Publishing Company., 2003)

Does God Laugh?
(Traverse City, Michigan: BMS Publications, 2008)

More information about Dr. Harvey and ordering information for the publications above are found at the web site:

www.sentencesermons.com

Breinigsville, PA USA
01 April 2010
235390BV00003B/23/P